NUTRITION, HYPERTENSION & CARDIOVASCULAR DISEASE SECOND EDITION

Ronald S. Smith

The Lyncean Press

Portland, Oregon

ISBN   0-9614229-1-2

CONTENTS

1. INTRODUCTION and PROSTAGLANDINS

This is the only book of its kind. For the first time all the important topics on nutrition, as they relate to hypertension and cardiovascular disease (CVD), are discussed in one volume. The information in this text comes directly from scientific journals and monographs. The scientific literature on many of these topics is extensive and often times conflicting. Every effort has been made to present a balanced, complete and up to date picture of each subject.

Each chapter or topic can be read independent of the others. A reader could easily start with the relationship of alcohol to hypertension in Chapter 16, then go back to fiber in Chapter 9, and then skip to potassium in Chapter 13. Chapters 1 and 2 are the most difficult, but they do provide some material that is useful in succeeding chapters.

In order to fit this much information into one volume, the writing, by necessity, is direct and compact. There is no fluff or filler material, no wasted words, sentences or paragraphs. There are many instances where a few pages contain as much useful information as a whole book. For example, the section on fiber covers oat bran and water soluble fiber in a few pages and the chapter on potassium is

9 pages long. There are popular books available that stretch each one of these topics out to several hundred pages.

CARDIOVASCULAR DISEASE (CVD)

Cardiovascular disease, which includes coronary heart disease (CHD), stroke and peripheral vascular disease, is the number one cause of death in the United States. There are almost one million CVD deaths per year compared to 460,000 for the second leading cause of death, cancer. The total cost for CVD in 1988 is estimated to be 84 billion dollars. The CVD death rate rose steadily through most of this century until the 1960's, when it leveled off and then began declining. Since 1968 the CVD death rate (on an age adjusted basis) has been declining between two and three percent per year. From 1968 to 1985, the rate declined a remarkable 35%. Nobody is sure why we are experiencing the decline. Some possible factors are: more exercise, improved detection and treatment, better diets along with certain dietary supplements, and less smoking. All of these topics are important, but it is beyond the scope of this book to discuss subjects other than the nutrition-cardiovascular disease link.

ATHEROSCLEROSIS

These short sections on atherosclerosis and prostaglandins will hopefully make some of the succeeding material on nutrients more meaningful. In the appendix is a brief unit on theories of the development of atherosclerosis.

Atherosclerosis is a condition found in almost all people having CVD. It is considered the principal cause of death in the U.S. and Western societies. The veins are rarely affected by this slowly developing disease, leaving the arteries as the usual site for atherosclerosis. Arterial disease, primarily atherosclerosis, is unquestionably the most important and costly disease in the Western world.

Arteries are composed of three main layers: the intima, the media and the adventitia. The intima, lining the inside of the artery, is the thinnest of the three. It is composed of a single sheet of endothelial cells supported by several types of connective tissue, including a sheet of porous elastin, called the internal elastic lamina. The intima is the primary site for atherosclerosis.

The <u>media</u> is made of connective tissue and smooth muscle cells, forming a muscular tube around the intima. In the larger arteries, such as the aorta or coronary artery, there are extra elastic fibers giving the vessel added strength.

The outermost layer is the <u>adventitia</u>. It contains various connective tissues, smooth muscle cells, arterioles (the vasa vasorium), lymphatic vessels and autonomic nerves. The vasa vasorium supplies the adventitia and the outer 2/3rds of the media with blood. The intima and inner part of the media are not supplied with blood by the vasa vasorium. They depend on oxygen and nutrients diffusing outward from blood in the lumen of the artery. If the intima thickens substantially, which occurs during atherosclerosis, part of the media will suffer from inadequate oxygen supply because the thickened intima will block its transport.

Atherosclerosis is the fundamental pathological process in CVD. It is a complex disease affecting arteries, characterized by greatly thickened intima and raised, lipid filled fibrous lesions. The term athero means gruel, which describes the viscous, fat and cholesterol rich material inside the lesion. Sclerosis refers to the fibrous hardening of the lesions. There are two lesion types found in arteries: <u>fatty streak</u>, and <u>fibrous plaque</u>. Fatty streak appears to be a normal occurance in humans. Fibrous plaque is the main lesion of atherosclerosis.

FATTY STREAK

Autopsy studies on infants indicate about half of all infants develop fatty streaks by age one. They occur universally in humans by age 12 even in populations in which atherosclerosis is rare. Fatty streaks are present in most mammalian species although most species rarely display atherosclerosis. Also, the distribution of fatty streak in children does not correspond to the locations of atherosclerosis in adults. These observations have suggested to many scientists that fatty streak is not the parent of fibrous plaque.

Fatty streaks appear as yellowish plaques on the inner surface of the aorta. The lipid is concentrated inside enlarged cells called foam cells. There is no other significant change in the intima. It is not thickened, filled with connective tissue or smooth muscle cells. They do not impede blood flow or have other symptoms associated with them. Fatty streaks are naturally occuring, non-pathological lesions. It is possible fatty streak represents the beginning of atherosclerosis, but there is also some scientific evidence indicating fatty streak may not be the starting point of atherosclerosis.

FIBROUS PLAQUE

Fibrous plaque is strikingly different than fatty streak. The intima is greatly thickened with connective tissue, macrophages and smooth muscle cells. The lesion is elevated above the intima, protruding into the lumen of the artery. Fibrous plaque has a white connective tissue 'cap' covering a pool of viscous lipids and cellular debris. The white covering gives the lesion its characteristic 'pearly' appearance. If an incision is made through the pearly cap, the yellow lipid gruel flows out.

The thickened intima contains proliferated smooth muscle cells which migrated from the media. The smooth muscle cells produce the excessive connective tissue found in the thickened intima. The tissue beneath the fibrous plaque suffers from various degrees of oxygen deprivation (hypoxia) because the diffusion of oxygen is impeded by the plaque. The hypoxia may account for the thinning of the tissue under the plaque and the dead tissue found in the lesion.

The oxygen deficit stimulates capillary growth from the arterioles in the outer layer of the artery. Because of this, advanced lesions are often well vascularized, which can lead to subsequent hemmorrhage. In addition, cellular debris, along with inflamation and leucocyte infiltration is a common finding in fibrous plaque. All of this paints a picture of a complex, pathological process.

As the plaque grows, protruding further into the arterial lumen, chronic oxygen deprivation can occur in the organs fed by the diseased vessels. When fibrous plaque occurs in the coronary artery, the condition is called coronary heart disease (CHD) or ischemic heart disease (IHD). Another insidious process is the thinning and softening of the connective tissue cap of the lesion, which can rupture, spilling out viscous fluid and precipitating a lethal clot.

Calcification occurs in older, more advanced plaque. The mechanism of calcification in the evolution of the lesion is not well understood. It is thought hypoxia promotes calcification. Once calcified, the lesion may crack, forming an ulcer and leaking out material which triggers clot formation.

PROSTAGLANDINS

Prostaglandins were first discovered in the prostate gland more than 45 years ago. It was many years before there was general interest in their important functions and properties. Almost all cells in the body either make or are affected by prostaglandins. There are over 20 prostaglandins made by cells, different cells making different ones. They are short lived (seconds rather than hours or days) hormone like substances with a variety of physiological effects, depending on the individual prostaglandin and the target cell.

Prostaglandins are not stored in any cells or glands, but rather are made rapidly when there is a need for them. Since they are not stored and have very short lifetimes, their cellular concentrations at any one time are extremely small. The small concentrations greatly inhibited interest in and understanding of the prostaglandins for many years because of the great difficulty in isolating, purifying and working with minute quantities of these compounds. Laboratory synthesis, which is done routinely now, was a great boon for prostaglandin research. Laboratory synthesis of prostaglandins has made it possible to do meaningful research on this important class of chemicals.

Prostaglandins are important for the cardiovascular system. Some prostaglandins promote atherosclerosis and CVD, while others help prevent the same. There is great interest in finding ways to increase the body's production of "good" prostaglandins and inhibit the production of the "bad" ones. There is evidence certain foods and nutrients increase the synthesis of "good" prostaglandins. In order to understand the importance of these nutrient effects, we need to be

aquainted with some of the prostaglandins, their sources and
properties.

One reason polyunsaturated fats (PUFA) are essential is
they are the starting materials for the manufacture of prostaglandins. Vegetable oils are excellent sources of PUFA.
The most common PUFA is linoleic acid. Linoleic acid is
needed to make many of the prostaglandins. The most important ones for the cardiovascular system made from linoleic
acid are Prostacyclin (PGI-2) and Thromboxane A-2 (TXA-2).

Thromboxane (TXA-2), a powerful inducer of platelet
aggregation, is made by the platelets. Platelet aggregation
is a key initial step in clot formation and release of other
chemicals by platelets, such as platelet derived growth
factor (PDGF) and serotonin. Serotonin raises blood pressure
by constricting blood vessels. PDGF causes smooth muscle
cells to migrate from the media to the intima. This is an
important first step in the development of atherosclerosis.
PDGF also stimulates the smooth muscle cells to proliferate
once they are in the intima. The evidence implicates PDGF as
a key promoter of atherosclerosis.

TXA-2 directly constricts blood vessels, thereby raising
blood pressure and reducing blood flow. There is now evidence of increased TXA-2 production in animals and humans
with diabetes or atherosclerosis. A vicious circle is set up,
whereby the increased TXA-2 causes platelets to release PDGF.
The PDGF promotes vascular disease and vascular disease
appears to promote increased TXA-2 production. In addition,
the TXA-2 and serotonin released by the platelets increase
blood pressure, which enhances atherosclerosis. From the
standpoint of CVD, TXA-2 would be considered a "bad" prostaglandin.

Prostacyclin (PGI-2) is made by the endothelium lining
blood vessels, heart and lung. PGI-2 is a powerful inhibitor
of platelet aggregation and platelet adherance to vessel
walls. PGI-2 also dilates blood vessels by relaxing smooth
muscle, thereby reducing blood pressure. By inhibiting
platelet aggregation and activation, PGI-2 prevents the
release of PDGF, the promoter of atherosclerosis. It also
prevents the formation of dangerous clots. The effects of
PGI-2 are in direct opposition to TXA-2, but it is important
to note, they are both made from the same polyunsaturated
fatty acid. Experimental work has demonstrated lower PGI-2

levels in both animals and humans with atherosclerosis and diabetes. From the standpoint of atherosclerosis, PGI-2 can be characterized as a "good" prostaglandin, an inhibitor of atherosclerosis, whereas TXA-2 is a "bad" prostaglandin, a promoter of atherosclerosis.

There are a number of drugs which inhibit prostaglandin production, the most common being aspirin and the non-steroidal anti-inflamatory compounds. At high doses of aspirin (1 to 3 per day) production of both PGI-2 and TXA-2 are inhibited with no benefit shown in controlled clinical trials of coronary artery disease patients. At lower doses of aspirin (1/7th to 1/2 aspirin every one to three days), the "bad" prostaglandin, TXA-2, is inhibited but the "good" one, PGI-2, is not inhibited. There is now good clinical evidence to demonstrate that low dose aspirin benefits patients with documented coronary artery disease and cerebral vascular disease.

Anturane (sulfinpyrazone), a relatively new drug, inhibits platelet aggregation and production of TXA-2. Large controlled trials using Anturane have claimed a 50% reduction in deaths during the first year after a heart attack in heart disease patients. These results suggest reduction of TXA-2 and platelet aggregation produces striking benefits in the cardiovascular system.

Peroxidized fats on the other hand, retard the production of the "good" prostaglandin, PGI-2. Fat peroxides accumulate in fibrous plaque and may be one of the reasons for reduced PGI-2 concentrations in humans and animals with atherosclerosis. Fat peroxides are found in oils used for deep frying and in deep fried foods. This is one reason to avoid routine consumption of french fried foods. Lipid peroxides are also endogenously produced. Vitamin E and other anti-oxidants block the peroxidation of lipids. There is now greater interest in vitamin E because of its potential effect on PGI-2 levels. Indeed, animal work has shown increased PGI-2 with vitamin E supplements and reduced PGI-2 during vitamin E deficiency.

Cigarette smoking affects PGI-2 production and platelet sensitivity to PGI-2. The umbilical arteries from babies of smoking mothers had markedly reduced PGI-2 concentrations. When the endothelial cells of the umbilical arteries were cultured, the cells from smoking mothers continued to produce

less PGI-2. Work on rat aorta shows nicotine retards PGI-2
production. A recent experiment on humans exposed to second
hand smoke strongly suggests passive smoking does have a
negative effect on PGI-2 function.

PROSTAGLANDIN THERAPY

Intravenous administration of "good" prostaglandins in
a number of vascular disease states has been studied and
reported. One of the first trials administered PGE-1 (a good
prostaglandin) intravenously to 37 advanced (facing amputation) peripheral vascular disease patients. Almost all of
the patients experienced complete relief of pain, remarkable
healing of ischemic ulcers and improved blood flow to the
extremities.

PgI-2 has been used with equally impressive results. A
short term study on five advanced peripheral vascular disease
patients using PGI-2, reported ischemic ulcer healing, regression of necrotic tissue and relief of resting pain. A
longer study, up to 15 months, using 30 advanced patients
showed only 40% of the patients had significant long term
improvement, although 80% had shorter improvement lasting up
to 2 months. A double blind trial using PGI-2 on Raynauds
syndrome patients reported good results also.

Only limited short term work has been done on coronary
artery disease patients. In animals with acute myocardial
ischemia, PGI-2 administration reduced infarct size, mortality, and myocardial oxygen demand. There is now good
human evidence to show PGI-2 infusions limit the amount of
heart damage during a heart attack. An interesting experiment was also done on open heart surgery patients using PGI-2
during the surgery. A reduction in platelet aggregation and
heparin requirement was documented during surgery, but most
important, a 50% decrease in bleeding after surgery was
noted.

The impressive benefits of prostaglandin therapy for
peripheral vascular disease strongly suggests prostaglandins
play a very important role in the health of the vascular
system. Any substance, by virtue of a 72 hour intravenous
drip, that can almost completely reverse a condition which
takes many years to develop, very likely is an integral part
of the health of the cardiovascular system.

REFERENCES

STATISTICS and ATHEROSCLEROSIS

Anonymous, Heart Facts.   American Heart Assn. 1988

Levy, Robert Declining mortality in coronary heart disease.
Arteriosclerosis 1:312-325,1981.

Mitchinson, M. & Ball, R.   Macrophages and atherogenesis
Lancet 2:146-49, 1987.

Ross, R. The pathogenesis of atherosclerosis- an update.
N Engl J Med 314:488-500, 1986

Ross, R. Platelet-derived growth factor. Ann Rev Med 38:
71-79, 1987.

PROSTAGLANDINS

Anonymous, Aspirin:what dose? Lancet 1:592-3, 1986.

Anonymous, Prostacyclin in therapuetics. Lancet 1:643, 1981.

Belch, J. et.al. Intermittent epoprostenol(PGI-2) infusion in
Raynaud's syndrome patients. Lancet 1:313-9, 1983.

Busacca, M. et.al. Reduced prostacyclin production by cultured endothelial cells from umbilical arteries of babies born
to women who smoke. Lancet 2:609-610, 1982.

Edlund, A. et. al. Myocardial ischaemia triggers formation of
TXA-2.   Lancet 2:573, 1987.

Green, K. et. al. Deficient PGI-2 formation after acute
myocardial infarction. Lancet 1:1037-8, 1987.

Henriksson, P. et. al. Limitation of MI with PGI-2.   in
Prostacyclin-Clinical Trials. Gryglewski, R. ed.   Raven
Press, New York, 1985.

Longmore, D. et.al. PGI-2n administration during cardiopulmonary bypass in man. Lancet 1:800-4, 1981.

McGiff J. TXA-2 & PGI-2: implications for function & disease of the vasculature. Adv Int Med 25:199-216, 1980.

Szczeklik, A. et.al. Successful therapy of advanced arteriosclerosis obliterans with PGI-2. Lancet 1:1111-4, 1979.

Szczeklik, A. et.al. PGI-2 therapy in peripheral arterial disease. Thrombosis Research 19:191-9, 1980.

2. LIPIDS: FAT, CHOLESTEROL and FISH OILS

A lipid is any water insoluble molecule made by a living organism. Both fat and cholesterol are lipids because they are water insoluble. Another name for fat is triglyceride. Triglycerides are usually classified according to the number of double bonds in the carbon chain. Saturated fats have no double bonds, monounsaturated fats have one double bond and polyunsaturated fats have two or more double bonds. Mono and polyunsaturated fats have never been implicated as causes of cardiovascular disease (CVD). There is research, which we will look at later, suggesting some of the polyunsaturated fats may be protective factors.

Excessive dietary saturated fat and cholesterol have been blamed for our epidemic of cardiovascular disease for decades. It is based on a long history of animal experimentation, human epidemiology and clinical trials. Elevated serum fat and cholesterol levels are well documented risk factors. Both of these risk factors are moderately raised by dietary saturated fat and cholesterol. In addition, human fibrous plaque usually contains excessive fat and cholesterol.

RISK FACTORS

There are many CVD risk factors. One researcher has tabulated 246 risk factors. Some of the common ones are weight, serum cholesterol, serum LDL and HDL, blood pressure, smoking, heredity and where you live. The primary strategy

in the diet prevention trials has been risk factor intervention, notably serum cholesterol reduction. In the United
States, the ideal serum cholesterol for males is between 130
and 190 mg%, with equal risk for any value within that range.
Men with serum cholesterol above 268 mg% are at twice the
risk compared to men with serum cholesterol between 130 and
190 mg%. Men with serum cholesterol above 240 mg% are
normally advised to attempt to lower their number.

The thirty year follow-up from the Framingham Study
revealed the surprising fact that serum cholesterol levels
after age 50 did not influence mortality. This shows that it
is more important to measure serum cholesterol at a young age
rather than old age. Also, there is a good deal of error in
individual cholesterol values. Many experts recommend 2 or 3
measurements be averaged.

LIPOPROTEINS

Lipids are not soluble in water, so they have to be
complexed with other materials in order to be transported by
blood. To overcome the solubility problem, various proteins
(called apoproteins), made by the liver and small intestine,
are combined with the lipids to make them water soluble. The
lipid-protein packets are called lipoproteins. The many
different lipoproteins are classified according to density.
The density classes of lipoproteins are: very low density
lipoprotein (VLDL); intermediate density lipoprotein (IDL);
low density lipoprotein (LDL) and high density lipoprotein
(HDL). LDL contains much more lipid than HDL, in fact, there
is so little fat and cholesterol carried by HDL that few
cardiologists paid attention to it until Miller and Miller's
historic paper in 1975.

Miller and Miller brought impressive epidemiological
evidence together to demonstrate elevated HDL protected
against CVD and a reduced level of HDL was a risk factor.
Many large studies support HDL's protective role, including
the Framingham, Tromso, and massive Co-operative Lipoprotein
Phenotyping studies.

There is now considerable evidence to show HDL carries
cholesterol from peripheral tissue back to the liver for
degradation and excretion. This is an important mechanism,

since ordinary cells cannot remove, degrade or excrete cholesterol. Once cholesterol invades arterial wall, the only way to remove it is to have it transported back to the liver by HDL. HDL is currently recognized as a powerful protective factor with greater risk predictive value than serum cholesterol. The large surveys indicate persons with HDL below 25 mg% have greater risk and persons above 45 mg% have much lower risk.

Low density lipoprotein (LDL) has the opposite relationship to heart disease. LDL correlates directly with CVD risk, appears to accelerate atherosclerosis and contains much more fat and cholesterol than HDL. LDL transports lipids from the liver to peripheral tissues including arterial wall. Most of the cholesterol in atherosclerotic lesions comes from LDL. Serum cholesterol (the amount of cholesterol found in all the lipoproteins) is usually elevated when LDL is elevated. The majority of studies indicate persons with LDL above 160 mg% have increased risk and persons below 130 mg% have reduced risk.

Diets with altered fat content primarily effect total serum cholesterol and LDL but not HDL. Reducing dietary cholesterol and saturated fat modestly lowers total serum cholesterol and LDL. Increasing dietary polyunsaturated fats modestly lowers total serum cholesterol and LDL also. We will see later that there is some evidence exercise, fish oils, alcohol, vitamins C and E elevate the protective HDL.

SATURATED FAT AND CHOLESTEROL

Animals vary in their response to dietary lipids. Rabbits and primates are the most sensitive. Vascular disease which is similar to human atherosclerosis can be produced in these animals by feeding them excessive saturated fat and cholesterol. Dogs, rats and mice are less sensitive to excessive saturated fat and cholesterol. These animals require high levels of vitamin D and blockade of thyroid hormone production, in addition to cholesterol and saturated fat, to induce atherosclerosis. The requirement of excessive vitamin D and inhibition of thyroid hormone production indicates atherosclerosis has a complex etiology.

The lipid rich diets designed to promote atherosclerosis usually contain casein, cellulose, sucrose and a vitamin mineral mix as the other ingredients. Many experiments have shown casein, cellulose and sucrose increase the ability of saturated fat and cholesterol to induce atherosclerosis. Replacing casein, cellulose and sucrose with soy protein, fiber and complex carbohydrates reduces and sometimes eliminates lipid induced vascular disease. This suggests lipids interact with other dietary factors to produce atherosclerosis. The animal experiments indicate dietary saturated fat and cholesterol are two of many dietary factors promoting atherosclerosis.

OXIDIZED CHOLESTEROL

The first experiments demonstrating dietary cholesterol induced vascular lesions in animals were reported in 1912. Between 1912 and 1975 a number of unresolved discrepancies were generated by inconsistent experimental results. One nagging problem was the severity of the induced atherosclerosis often depended on the method of raising the serum cholesterol. In 1956 the eminent organic chemist, Louis Fieser, suggested some of the cholesterol in the feeding trials was being oxidized during the mixing of the feed, thereby adding unknown compounds which may be influencing the experimental atherosclerosis.

In 1976 Imai et. al. resolved this problem by concentrating the oxidized impurities found in USP cholesterol and feeding the impurities to rabbits. The rabbits given the oxidized cholesterol orally had a much higher incidence of degenerated aortic cells and aortic cell debris after 24 hours than those fed purified cholesterol. Vascular lesions remarkably similar to man's occured in rabbits 7 weeks after repeated administration of the oxidized cholesterol. Lesions were not found in animals repeatedly given purified cholesterol.

Taylor et. al. in 1979 confirmed and extended these startling findings. They reported the fresh USP cholesterol bottle they were using contained 5% oxidation products and a 5 year old jar was contaminated with an amazing 40% oxidized cholesterol. The concentrated impurities applied at a dosage 1/100th the amount of purified USP cholesterol used, produced

5 times the cellular debris as the purified cholesterol. Using these numbers, they suggest oxidized cholesterol is 500 times more damaging than pure cholesterol. More recent intravenous experiments have confirmed the oral studies, that is, oxidized cholesterol damages endothelium and smooth muscle cells, but pure cholesterol does not. Taylor et. al. separated the various impurities and found 25-hydroxycholesterol was the most angiotoxic oxidized steroid. Other workers have reported 25-hydroxycholesterol and similar oxidation products occur in human atherosclerotic lesions. Taylor et. al. concluded their important review by saying, "It would appear that nearly all of the studies on the induction of atherosclerosis by feeding USP cholesterol stored in air at room temperature should be reevaluated. The cholesterol used in experimental diets, in the majority of instances, probably contained significant quantities of oxidized sterols that have a strikingly lethal effect on aortic smooth muscle cells."

Most foods have not been analyzed yet for oxidized cholesterol. Any food containing cholesterol exposed to heat and air for extended periods of time is suspect. Powdered whole egg or egg yolk and powdered whole milk have been analyzed and do contain oxidized cholesterol. When a food is spray dried, which is the common method of powdering eggs and milk, the perfect conditions for cholesterol oxidation are met, because the food is intimately mixed with heat and air until dry. It seems reasonable to avoid powdered egg and powdered whole milk or any prepared food containing them. Dried whey, cheeses stored at room temperature, a powdered custard mix, a pancake mix containing whole egg solids and lard used for deep frying, on analysis, contained oxidized cholesterol. Foods suspected but not proven to contain oxidized cholesterol are smoked fish and meat, especially if stored at room temperature, some cheeses, and evaporated whole milk.

Recently it was shown Indian Ghee (specially clarified butter) contains 12% cholesterol oxides whereas ordinary butter does not. Johnson suggested the unexpectedly high rate of CVD amongst immigrants from India living in London is due to their use of Ghee, which contains 12% oxidized cholesterol.

Egg yolks, since they are the most concentrated source of cholesterol (250 mg per yolk), deserve special mention. The early experiments using egg yolk to induce atherosclerosis very likely contained oxidized cholesterol due to their use of powdered egg yolk. Fresh eggs very likely do not contain oxidized cholesterol since there are no reports claiming they do. Animal experiments in 1958 and common sense suggest soft boiling is the safest way to prepare eggs. The more heat and air eggs are exposed to during preparation, the greater the likelihood of oxidation, but unfortunately, eggs prepared by different methods have not been analysed.

RECOMMENDATIONS: OXIDIZED CHOLESTEROL

The potent vessel damaging properties of oxidized cholesterol is a very important, but neglected, discovery. There is an urgent need to analyse common foods for oxidized cholesterol. It is known powdered egg yolk, powdered whole milk and Indian Ghee (clarified butter) contain oxidized cholesterol. It would be wise to avoid these substances alone or in prepared foods.

Eggs are singled out here because egg yolks contain more cholesterol than any other common food. Fresh eggs very likely do not contain oxidized cholesterol. Most experts advise against excessive egg consumption because of their high cholesterol content and not because of oxidized cholesterol. Products containing powdered or dried egg do contain oxidized cholesterol and should be avoided.

EPIDEMIOLOGY:SATURATED FAT & CHOLESTEROL

Many international surveys have clearly demonstrated a significant correlation between a country's average saturated fat consumption and its CVD death rate. The same holds true for cholesterol consumption and CVD death rate. Nations with excessive cholesterol and saturated fat diets have very high rates of CVD. This of course is not proof that lipids are the cause of the high rates, but it does support the animal findings.

Interestingly, there are certain kinds of surveys which do not fit the fat-CVD hypothesis. For example, almost all surveys of populations within one country have not demonstrated a relationship between dietary saturated fat and CVD or between dietary cholesterol and CVD. The Framingham study did not find a difference in total fat, saturated fat or cholesterol consumption for persons who developed CVD compared to those who did not. The same lack of expected relationship was found in the 7200 man Honolulu Heart Study and the 8200 man Puerto Rico survey.

A recent analysis of 62,000 deaths in Iowa men shows a more contrary pattern. Iowa farmers had significantly lower CVD death rates than nonfarmers, but the farmers consumed 25% more cholesterol and 10% more saturated fat than the non-farm men. These results stand in clear opposition to the lipid- heart hypothesis. In a four year study of 2,000 Michigan men, Paul et.al. found no association between dietary cholesterol and development of CVD. The surprising lack of relationship between lipid intake and CVD death rate within one area or country suggests there are probably many dietary factors involved in CVD in addition to saturated fat and cholesterol.

SERUM CHOLESTEROL

Animals put on high saturated fat and cholesterol diets respond with serum cholesterol elevations. In human controlled trials, where cholesterol and saturated fat are added to the diet, serum cholesterol rises moderately. When cholesterol and saturated fat are removed from the diet, serum cholesterol falls moderately. The large scale prevention trials, where saturated fat and cholesterol consumption were reduced, there was an average 10% drop in serum cholesterol. There is usually a great variability in individual response.

Internationally, there is a significant relationship between saturated fat or cholesterol consumption and serum cholesterol levels, but for groups within one country, serum cholesterol doesn't seem to be linked to dietary cholesterol or saturated fat. The Framingham Study, for instance, found serum cholesterol to be independent of dietary lipids in that free living group of people. An investigation of 10,000 Israeli men found the same independence. The Tecumseh Study of 2,000 subjects reported no correlation between dietary lipids and serum cholesterol. The surprising lack of relationship suggests there are other factors affecting serum cholesterol in addition to dietary cholesterol and saturated fat. In this book we will look at several other food factors affecting serum cholesterol.

All saturated fats are normally thought to raise serum cholesterol. This apparently is not true. Bonanome and Grundy recently reconfirmed some previous neglected work which demonstrated stearic acid actually lowers serum cholesterol in humans. Stearic acid is an 18 carbon saturated fatty acid found in animal fat, including beef, and in chocolate. Certainly information like this makes the whole issue of saturated fat confusing. It is beyond the intended scope of this book to enter the complex debate on dietary cholesterol, saturated fat and CVD. Readers interested in this fascinating and never ending debate should consult the following provocative papers: Ahrens (1985), Stehbens (1987), Raymond (1988), Gorringe (1986) and McGill (1979).

HISTORICAL PATTERNS

The historical food consumption patterns in the United States do not fit well with the lipid-heart hypothesis. From 1909 to 1961, a period of enormous increase in coronary heart disease, the changes in saturated fat and cholesterol intakes were trivial. Cholesterol and saturated fat increased about 7% in that time period. The greatest changes in food consumption patterns were the substantial decreases in flour, cereal, potato and complex carbohydrates along with the substantial increase in polyunsaturated fats and a moderate increase in simple sugars.

PREVENTION TRIALS

Altering fat consumption is the only dietary strategy tested so far in controlled trials to prevent CVD. None of the controlled trials were low in total fat, but instead were low in saturated fat and cholesterol and moderately rich in polyunsaturated fat. The first experiments in the 1950's and early 1960's were poorly controlled but did report encouraging results. The later experiments were better controlled but the results were disappointing. At present none of the well controlled trials have convincingly demonstrated lower CVD death rates. They have reported reduced serum cholesterol and a trend towards declining death rate, but not a statistically significant trend. On balance, the prevention trials, utilizing changes in dietary fat, have been failures. The fact that they have been failures does not mean saturated fat and dietary cholesterol have nothing to do with the disease. It probably means these diet factors play a smaller role than is generally assumed. The reader should also be reminded that CVD is a slow, silent disease that could well take thirty years to fully develop. Hence a definitive prevention trial should last 20 or 30 years. The longest of the diet prevention trials has only been 5 years.

Prevention trials using drugs to lower serum cholesterol have had their share of disappointment also. Except for the the experiment reported in January, 1984, none of the serum cholesterol lowering drugs have reduced death rates in CVD patients. In 1984 the Lipid Research Clinics Coronary Primary Prevention Trial results, using cholestryamine resin to reduce serum cholesterol, were published. This well designed, lengthy (9 years) and expensive ($120,000,000) trial was the first to conclusively demonstrate that reducing serum cholesterol in persons with hypercholesterolemia will lower their death rate from CVD. The results on the 3806 men were self consistent, that is, the lowest death rates occured in the groups with the greatest fall in serum cholesterol, so there was a great probability the effect was real. These results strongly suggest reducing serum cholesterol by any means, whether it be diet, exercise or drugs, will lower CVD death rate.

SUMMARY and RECOMMENDATIONS:
SATURATED FAT and CHOLESTEROL

Animal and human evidence exists implicating dietary cholesterol and saturated fat as promoters of atherosclerosis and CVD, but the evidence is not as consistent or strong as generally assumed. Lowering dietary cholesterol, saturated fat and total fat consumption appears to be a wise thing to do. This change has never been shown to be harmful. Serum cholesterol, triglycerides, LDL and weight will be reduced somewhat by controlling fat intake. In addition, a low lipid diet allows much more room for fiber, complex carbohydrates, and high nutrient foods such as vegetables, legumes, whole grains and fruits.

The American Heart Association recommends no more than 30% of our calories be from fat, with a maximum of 10% from saturated fat and 300 mg of cholesterol. A 20% fat diet would be better (and is recommended by the AHA for CVD patients), allowing more room for protective foods. Severe limitations on concentrated fats, such as, oil, margarine, butter, mayonnaise, salad dressing, cheese, pasteries and fatty meats would bring most people down to a 20% fat diet. In the next section we will discuss individual lipids, their dietary sources and properties.

CHOLESTEROL

The source of cholesterol is both diet and the liver. The liver can use carbohydrate, fat or protein to synthesize cholesterol. The liver's ability to make cholesterol is an important function to keep in mind when you try to resolve the imperfect relationship between dietary cholesterol and serum cholesterol. Each person's liver is an uncontrollable variable, linking, often in an unpredictable fashion, dietary cholesterol and serum cholesterol. This is not to say dietary intake and serum levels have no relationship. There is a link, but it is not always very predictable.

All animals make cholesterol, whether they be worms, ants, cows or humans. Plants do not make cholesterol (this is why vegetable oils never contain cholesterol). Mammals use it for cell membrane structure, to make steroid hormones (estrogen, progesterone, corticol, testosterone etc.), cholic acid (an important component of bile), lanolin, vitamin D and myelin, which is necessary for nerve axons. Cholesterol is essential for mammals.

A 150 pound man contains about one third of a pound of cholesterol (140,000 mg). On a dry weight basis, one third of a pound amounts to almost 1% of the bodies dry mass, an unusually large percentage for one compound. In the blood, only sodium chloride and a few proteins occur in larger amounts. Even though only 7% of the total body cholesterol is found in the blood, there is more of it in the blood of a normal healthy person than glucose.

The human liver makes between 1,000 mg and 1,600 mg of cholesterol per day. When dietary cholesterol goes up, the liver compensates by producing less. The average American consumes about 500 to 600 mg daily, but less than half of this is absorbed. Egg yolk, containing about 250 mg of cholesterol, provides more than any other common food. Greatly restricting eggs is the surest way to reduce dietary cholesterol to the American Heart Associations recommended maximum of 300 mg. The following is the cholesterol content of some selected foods:

Cream, 1 oz	20 mg
Cottage Cheese, 1/2 cup	24 mg
Ice Cream, 1/2 cup	27 mg
Cheddar Cheese, 1 oz	28 mg
Whole Milk, 1 cup	34 mg
Lard, 1 tablespoon	12 mg
Butter, 1 tablespoon	35 mg
Oysters, salmon, 3 oz	40 mg
Clams, tuna, 3 oz	55 mg
Beef, Pork, Lobster, Chicken, Turkey, 3 oz	75 mg
Lamb, veal, crab, 3 oz	85 mg
Shrimp, 3 oz	130 mg
Beef Heart, 3 oz	230 mg
Egg, one yolk	250 mg
Liver, 3 oz	370 mg
Kidney, 3 oz	680 mg
Brains, 3 oz	1700 mg

ANIMAL AND VEGETABLE FATS

Vegetable fats do not contain cholesterol but all animal fats do. Nevertheless, selecting fats on the basis of animal versus vegetable is not the best method, because some vegetable oils are better than others and some animal fats are beneficial. Palm oil and coconut oil, for instance, are rich in palmitic acid, a saturated fat which raises serum cholesterol. Rapeseed oil, although not rich in saturated fat, if it contains eurucic acid, causes heart muscle damage in animals. Fish oils, on the other hand, have remarkable protective properties, even though they are classified as animal fats.

About 38% of the calories in the average American diet comes from fat. For the average 2400 calorie diet, this means 900 calories are from fat. The following table lists the percentage and number of fat colories in some common foods:

Food	Per Cent Fat	Fat Calories
Butter, 1 tbs	100% fat	100
Margarine, 1 tbs	100% fat	100
Salad oil, 1 tbs	100% fat	120
Mayonnaise, 1 tbs	100% fat	100
Salad Dressing, 1 tbs	85% fat	65
Beef, lean, 3 oz	33% fat	55
Beef, not lean, 3 oz	55% fat	145
Bacon, crisp, 4 slices	85% fat	145
Link Sausage, 3 links	90% fat	160
Ham, 3 0z	70% fat	170
Pork chop, lean, 3 oz	55% fat	120
Pork chop, not lean, 3 oz	75% fat	250
Bologna, 3 slices	85% fat	210
Almonds, 2 oz	80% fat	280
Peanuts, 2 oz	75% fat	270
Milk Chocolate, 2 oz	55% fat	160
Cookies, 2 oz,	40% fat	100
Cheese, cheddar, 1 oz	70% fat	80
Milk, whole, 1 cup	50% fat	75
Ice Cream, 1 cup	45% fat	125
Egg, 1 whole	65% fat	55
Beans, 1/2 cup	5% fat	5
Bread, 2 slices	10% fat	15
Fruits	trace	trace
Vegetables	trace	trace

SATURATED FAT

Saturated fats do not contain unsaturated bonds, which chemists call double bonds. Saturated fats can be synthesized by the liver and other tissues from carbohydrate, protein or fat. If you avoid all saturated fat your tissues will make some for you. All vegetable and animal fats contain saturated fat, but animal sources have 2 to 4 times more.

The American Heart Association recommends no more than 10% of the calories be from saturated fat. If the average person consumes a total of 2400 calories per day, then 10% is 240 calories. Fat has 9 calories per gram, so the American Heart Association is recommending a maximum of 26 grams (a little less than one ounce) of saturated fat. Diet surveys have reported an average range of 38 to 48 grams for Americans. In order to get below the AHA maximum, the average American needs to reduce saturated fat by 15 to 20 grams per day.

Dairy fat, luncheon meats, sausage, organ meats, fatty meats and milk chocolate are unusually rich in saturated fat. Restricting these foods would put most people below 10% saturated fat and leave plenty of room for low fat, nutrient rich foods, such as, vegetables, fruit, legumes, cereals, and fish. The following is the saturated fat content of some selected foods:

Cheddar Cheese, 1 oz	6.1 grams
Whole Milk, 1 cup	5.8 grams
Evaporated Milk, 1 cup	11.5 grams
Eggnog, 1 cup	11.5 grams
Ice Cream, 1 cup	9.0 grams
Egg, 1 whole	1.7 grams
Butter, 1 tbs	7.2 grams
Margarine, 1 tbs	2.1 grams
Lard, 1 tbs	5.1 grams
Salad oils, 1 tbs, ave	2.0 grams
Beef, very lean, 3 oz	2.0 grams
Beef, not lean, 3 oz	12.0 grams
Bologna, 3 slices	9.0 grams
Sausage, pork link, 3 oz	12.5 grams
Turkey, light meat, 3 oz	1.0 grams
Almonds, 1 oz	1.0 grams

Peanuts, 1 oz_____ 2.5 grams
Walnuts, 1 oz_____ 2.0 grams
Milk Chocolate, 2 oz_____ 11.0 grams
Whole wheat flour,_____ trace
Cooked beans,_____ trace
Peas, 1 cup_____ trace
Vegetables_____ trace
Fruit_____ trace

MONOUNSATURATED FAT

A monounsaturated fat has only one carbon-carbon double bond in its carbon chain. Oleic acid is the most common monounsaturated fat. It is not an essential fat because it can be synthesized by mammals, including humans. Under normal circumstances oleic acid is not converted into other fatty acids nor is it a starting material for prostaglandin production. It occurs in generous amounts in all lipid containing foods, whether animal or vegetable. Animal fats vary from 20 to 40% oleic acid and vegetable oils from 12% for safflower oil to 75% for olive oil.

For many years oleic acid was considered a neutral fat in terms of causing or preventing CVD, since it appeared to have little effect on serum cholesterol. There is good agreement oleic acid does not raise serum cholesterol. Furthermore, recent work by Mattson has reported a serum cholesterol lowering effect for oleic acid as great as for linoleic acid. Epidemiology of Europe has generated new interest in oleic acid due to countries like Italy and Greece where there is copious consumption of oleic acid and low rates of heart disease.

This new information on oleic acid has prompted some people to use very large amounts of olive oil to protect themselves against heart disease. It seems to this author it is premature to use olive oil as a medication, but certainly it can be used in reasonable amounts without much fear of it causing atherosclerosis. Olive oil is highly recommended for frying because it is not damaged by heat the way polyunsaturated oils are. It is also very expensive and flavorful, which tends to encourage people to use less, thereby they consume fewer empty calories.

POLYUNSATURATED FAT

Polyunsaturated fat contains fatty acids with two or more double bonds. Polyunsaturated fatty acids (PUFA) are considered essential because they cannot be made by mammals and because liver abnormalities and dermatitis develop when there is an inadequate supply. Prostaglandins cannot be manufactured without PUFA, which is another reason PUFA is essential.

There are two PUFA families. Linoleic acid, the most common PUFA, is the first member of the so called omega-6 fatty acid family. Linolenic acid is the first member of the omega-3 fatty acid family. Each family has different polyunsaturated fatty acids which are the starting materials for different prostaglandins. The figures on the next page show the members of each family along with the prostaglandin each fat makes.

OMEGA-6 FATTY ACIDS

Linoleic acid, the most common PUFA, is the parent of the omega-6 family. Symptoms of essential fatty acid deficiency develop when linoleic acid (or other PUFA) intake is less than 1 or 2 percent of total calories, which is equivalent to 2.5 to 5 grams daily. Above 5 grams of linoleic acid (or other PUFA) per day there is virtually no risk of developing essential fatty acid deficiency.

Linoleic acid is converted by the liver and other cells into dihomo-gamma-linolenic acid (DHLA). Except for evening primrose oil, few foods or plants contain this fatty acid. DHLA is the fatty acid required for the production of the beneficial prostaglandin PGE-1.

DHLA is changed by the liver and other cells into arachidonic acid. There are no dietary sources of arachidonic acid. It is the starting material for the beneficial PGI-2 and the harmful prostaglandin, TXA-2.

The hypocholesterolemic property of linoleic acid has been known for many years. It was the rationale for adding copious amounts of vegetable oils to the regimens of heart disease patients and to the protocols of prevention trials. It took large quantities oils rich in linoleic acid to reduce the serum cholesterol moderately. Prevention and treatment diets with 300 calories of vegetable oil added were common.

MEMBERS OF THE OMEGA-6 FAMILY

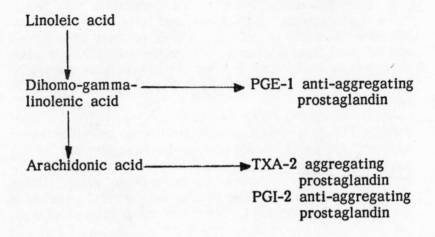

Linoleic acid

Dihomo-gamma-linolenic acid ⟶ PGE-1 anti-aggregating prostaglandin

Arachidonic acid ⟶ TXA-2 aggregating prostaglandin
PGI-2 anti-aggregating prostaglandin

MEMBERS OF THE OMEGA-3 FAMILY

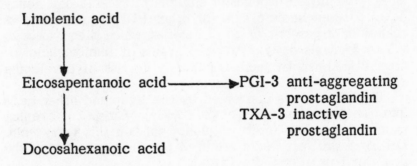

Linolenic acid

Eicosapentanoic acid ⟶ PGI-3 anti-aggregating prostaglandin
TXA-3 inactive prostaglandin

Docosahexanoic acid

For a decade or so, heart disease prevention was a game of eliminating saturated fats and loading up on linoleic acid. The poor results and poor compliance exhibited by the prevention trials along with the suspected side effects (weight gain, gall bladder disease, cancer) of salad oil diets, turned the tide against advocating oil rich diets. The American Heart Association has reduced their recommendation for linoleic acid. They suggest a maximum of 10% of the calories from PUFA, an amount found in three tablespoons of corn oil.

Ten percent linoleic acid is high by historical standards. Prior to the 20th century, most diets were 8 to 12% total fat, with only 4 to 8% of the calories from PUFA. Tissue analyses world wide have revealed linoleic acid consumption in the United States is similar to other populations. Large surveys have reported average diets in the United States contain 5 to 7% PUFA, the majority of which is linoleic acid. The American Heart Association recommends increasing that amount to 8 to 10% and sharply reducing saturated fats, a strategy which usually yields a 10% lowering in serum cholesterol.

There is some confusion on linoleic acids effect on serum triglyceride. Several short term experiments on healthy humans claimed moderate decreases in serum triglyceride whereas a number of longer experiments reported no effect. A similar variability in experimental response occurs when hyperlipidemic subjects are tested with linoleic acid. A high linoleic diet does not appear to be a promising prescription for the reduction of plasma triglyceride.

The plasma lipoproteins are effected by linoleic acid. When serum cholesterol is reduced, usually LDL goes down because the majority of the cholesterol in the plasma is carried by LDL. Linoleic acid administration follows this pattern of serum cholesterol and LDL reductions. Unfortunately, half the experiments on humans have reported reduction of the beneficial HDL also. There are no reports claiming elevation of HDL using linoleic acid. Until the divergent HDL responses to linoleic acid are resolved, caution towards excessive linoleic acid intake is warranted.

Feeding linoleic acid to animals or humans results in a reduction of platelet aggregation, but no increase in bleeding time. Reduction in platelet aggregation is a beneficial property because platelet aggregation and hyperactive platelets promotes atherosclerosis. A number of experiments on humans and animals have demonstrated increased ingestion of linoleic acid reduces the arachidonic acid content of platelets and endothelium. Production of TXA-2, the platelet aggregating prostaglandin, is reduced due the diminished arachidonic acid content of the platelets. This is the most likely reason for the reduced platelet aggregation with linoleic acid feeding.

A discouraging finding with excessive linoleic acid is the decrease in PGI-2 production by the endothelium. PGI-2 is a powerful inhibitor of platelet aggregation and appears to retard atherosclerosis. The decrease in PGI-2 production suggests there may be long term detrimental effects from excessive linoleic consumption which may negate the benefits of decreased platelet aggregation.

We mentioned above the minimum amount of linoleic acid needed to prevent essential fatty acid deficiency is 3 to 5 grams per day and the maximum recommended by the AHA is 26 grams daily. Animal fats do supply small amounts of linoleic acid. People eating generous amounts of beef, chicken or pork, dairy products will get between 2 and 3 grams from these sources. Fruits, vegetables, beans and grains contain very little fat. Bakery goods will supply linoleic acid if the recipe included salad oil. Vegetable oils, nuts and seeds are outstanding sources of linoleic acid. For example, three walnuts provides 5 grams of PUFA and will prevent essential fatty acid deficiency. The following are the amounts of linoleic acid found in one ounce of each food:

corn oil	16g	olive oil	2g
peanut oil	8g	safflower oil	20g
soybean oil	9g	regular margarine	6g
mayonnaise	11g	soft margarine	8g
almonds	3g	brazil nuts	14g
cashews	2g	peanuts	4g
pumpkin seeds	5g	sunflower seeds	9g
walnuts	11g	pecans	5g

Dihomo-gamma-linolenic acid (DHLA), a metabolite of linoleic acid, is not found in plant oils except for evening primrose oil. Feeding DHLA to animals or humans usually increases the platelet and endothelium concentration of DHLA. DHLA can be converted into arachidonic acid(the precursor to TXA-2 and PGI-2, the aggregating and anti-aggregating prostaglandins respectively) or into PGE-1, an important anti-aggregating prostaglandin. In theory, DHLA should increase the production of the beneficial PGE-1. This is why there is considerable interest in evening primrose oiL A few clinical investigations reported decreased platelet aggregation with oral DHLA, but others have not confirmed this effect. Several trials have reported serum cholesterol reduction with evening primrose oil. More clinical work needs to be done before recommendations on evening primrose supplements can be given.

SUMMARY AND RECOMMENDATIONS: LINOLEIC ACID

Prevention trials have not demonstrated excessive linoleic acid will lower death rate or prevent coronary heart disease. The effects of linoleic acid on risk factors are conflicting. Some risk factors are benefited and others are made worse. Since no clear benefit can be demonstrated, it seems to this author that the American Heart Association's recommendation of 10% linoleic acid is excessive. The National Research Council has determined 3% of the calories from linoleic acid (or PUFA) provides an adequate margin of safety. Three or four walnuts supplies this amount of PUFA. By limiting linoleic acid to 3 to 5% of the calories, there is more room left for high nutrient, protective foods.

OMEGA-3 FATTY ACID FAMILY

Persons seeing the world through lipid eyes would characterize the 1950's to the 1960's as the omega-6 era and the mid 1970's through the 1980's as the omega-3 era. There has been great excitement about eicosapentanoic acid (EPA), the fish oil member of omega-3. The parent fatty acid for the family is linolenic acid, also called alpha-linolenic acid. Linolenic acid is not the same molecule as dihomo-gamma-linolenic acid and they are not members of the same fatty acid family. Eicosapentanoic acid is the first and most important product of linolenic acid, at least in relation to CVD. Docosahexaenoic acid, produced from eicosapentanoic acid, is a much less important molecule for CVD, but it is extremely important in the central nervous system. One intriguing thing about the fats in the omega-3 family is they make beneficial prostaglandins exclusively, without making corresponding harmful ones.

LINOLENIC ACID

The interest in omega-3 fatty acids is focused around eicosapentanoic acid leaving the family parent, linolenic acid, rather neglected. Except for walnut oil (11% linolenic acid) there are few dietary sources of linolenic acid. Linseed oil contains a prodigious 55% linolenic acid, but it is not a common food. Soybean oil is 7% linolenic acid but partial hydrogenation removes most of it.

Feeding rats a diet containing 4% linolenic acid greatly increased the eicosapentanoic acid concentration of the serum and liver and significantly reduced serum cholesterol in both rats and chickens. The serum cholesterol reductions were greater than for linoleic acid.

There is a paucity of human work on linolenic acid. One experiment fed linseed oil to one volunteer and no increase in serum eicosapentanoic acid was reported. Platelet or endothelial concentrations were not measured. Another linseed oil trial reported no changes in platelet adhesiveness or bleeding times. There have been no long term investigations of prostaglandin production, platelet function, serum triglyceride or cholesterol response to linolenic acid administration. Eicosapentanoic acid greatly benefits the above parameters, so it seems reasonable linolenic acid would also since linolenic acid is converted into eicosapentanoic acid by most tissues. This likely possibility should be thoroughly researched.

Walnuts are interesting to consider as a source of PUFA. They are 88% fat on a caloric basis, and 66% of that fat is polyunsaturated, which is much higher than any of the other common nuts or seeds. The oils in almonds, for example, are only 18% polyunsaturated. The most unusual characteristic of walnuts is their high content of linolenic acid, whereas most other nuts have very little linolenic acid. Three walnuts provides six grams of essential fatty acids so a person on a low fat diet would be assured of avoiding essential fatty acid deficiency by eating three walnuts per day. The extra for walnuts is the theoretically beneficial linolenic acid it provides.

EICOSAPENTANOIC ACID (EPA)

There is some epidemiology on Greenland and Alaskan coastal Eskimos suggesting dietary eicosapentanoic acid (EPA) is responsible for their unusually low rate of CHD and atherosclerosis. Their low rate is particularly striking because of their rich animal fat diets. The key to their CVD health appeared to be the copious consumption of fish, whale and seal oils, all of which are unique in containing appreciable amounts of EPA. EPA rarely occurs in other sources of fat. Generous amounts of EPA, along with EPA's chief prostaglandin product, the anti-aggregating and arteriole dilating PGI-3, were found in the serum and platelets of Eskimos. The unique Eskimo epidemiology stimulated interest in fish oils and EPA.

ANIMAL STUDIES: EPA

A number of reports indicate EPA is more effective in reducing serum cholesterol and triglycerides in experimental animals than linoleic acid. EPA supplements also decrease the omega-6 series lipids (linoleic and arachidonic acid) and their corresponding prostaglandins (TXA-2 and PGI-2) in experimental animals. Limited work has shown reduced platelet aggregation and increased bleeding times after EPA administration. A series of important investigations by Culp et. al. revealed dogs given experimentally induced myocardial infarcts have significantly decreased infarct size (3% vs 25% of left ventricle) in animals pretreated with fish oil. Cats pretreated with fish oil had reduced brain damage (7% vs 19% of brain volume) following closure of the cerebral artery. Culp et. al. proposed three possible ways EPA reduced tissue damage after ischemia, namely: arteriole dilation; reduced constriction of microvasculature; and diminished microthrombi formation.

There is now convincing evidence from animals that fish oils prevent atherosclerosis. Pigs put on high cholesterol and saturated fat diets were protected against atherosclerosis by fish oil supplements. The fish oils were protective even though the animals serum cholesterol remained exceedingly high. Experiments on monkeys and dogs have shown similar powerful results.

HUMAN WORK: EPA

During the 1950's and 1960's eight fish oil studies were performed on humans without generating lasting interest. The fish oils were hypocholesterolemic but not noticibly more than linoleic acid. Since linoleic acid is cheaper and more convenient to administer, the fish oils were forgotten until the Eskimo epidemiology. Several important features of the early work were not appreciated. First, it took about two to five times less fish oil to lower serum cholesterol than linoleic acid. Second, the fish oil groups didn't have their dietary cholesterol controlled. In general the fish oil group had 300mg to 500mg greater cholesterol intake than the linoleic acid subjects, hence their serum cholesterol did not drop as much as it would have on a lower cholesterol diet. Third, serum triglyceride response was not measured, thereby not detecting the important and unique triglyceride lowering effect of fish oils.

In subjects with normal serum lipids given 20 to 29g of EPA per day, serum cholesterol was lowered 14%, triglycerides a remarkable 33%, and the atherogenic LDL, 16%. There were no changes in HDL. A comparable vegetable oil diet did not reduce serum triglycerides and had a less significant effect on LDL.

Hyperlipidemic patients have responded extremely well to EPA. One study reported fish oil rich diets reduced plasma cholesterol 31% and plasma triglyceride an astounding 66%. In 4 severely hyperlipidemic patients (plasma cholesterol= 347, plasma triglyceride= 1534) plasma cholesterol fell to 189 (a 46% drop) and triglycerides fell to 354mg% (a 77% drop) after 4 weeks on a 30% salmon oil diet in comparison to a 5% total fat diet previous to the salmon oil. After the salmon oil, the patients were put on a high linoleic acid-vegetable oil regimen, but the serum cholesterol and triglyceride levels began rising so rapidly, the vegetable oils had to be discontinued. Other studies, along with the above experiments, demonstrate a consistent pattern of dramatic triglyceride reduction and moderate cholesterol lowering.

Trials providing smaller quantities of EPA, in the range of 4 to 10 grams of EPA daily, show less consistent effects on serum cholesterol. Some reported non-significant effects on serum cholesterol, but all of them have claimed triglyceride reduction. One recent report by Fehily et. al. on 118 healthy men demonstrated a significant 7% fall in serum triglyceride after three months of adding one half pound of fatty fish per week to their diet. The added fish provided less than 1 gram of EPA per day. Another important consistent finding is the absence of HDL lowering, in fact, some trials claim HDL elevations. It should be remembered, one of the worrisome findings on linoleic acid vegetable oils is reduction in the beneficial HDL levels.

Another area of great excitement is EPA's reduction of platelet aggregation, decrease in the aggregating prostaglandin TXA-2, and increase in bleeding time. These effects have been demonstrated many times in normals and patients. One of the first experiments fed one to one and a half pounds of mackerel daily to 7 healthy men, which provided 7 to 11 grams of EPA. After 6 days, platelet aggregation decreased 50% when challenged with collagen while TXB-2 output decreased 30%. Thorngren and Gustafson had 10 healthy volunteers increase their fish consumption to provide 2 to 3 grams of EPA daily for 11 weeks. They had marked increase in EPA content of the platelets, a 42% increase in bleeding time and a pronounced decrease in platelet aggregation. Saynor and Verel gave 19 volunteers 1.8 or 3.6 grams of EPA in capsule form daily for 12 months. There was a 37% decrease in triglyceride but no increase in bleeding time for the 1.8 gram group. The 3.6 gram subjects had a 100% increase in bleeding time. These and other reports indicate 2 to 5 grams of EPA produces measureable and significant improvement in risk factors.

Harris et. al. gave 5, 8 or 13 grams of EPA per day to 11 hyperlipidemic patients. On the 5 gram dose, serum cholesterol went down 16% and triglycerides a remarkable 52%. On 13 grams the triglycerides decreased 63% and bleeding time increased 51%. Hay et. al. investigated platelet kinetics in CHD patients after taking 3.5 grams of EPA for 3 weeks. Improvement in platelet survival and various clotting factors were noted. These reports suggest low doses of EPA are strikingly beneficial in CVD patients.

There are many other exceedingly powerful effects of fish oils that have been reported. First, they prevent human endothlial cells from producing 'platelet derived growth factor like protein', a protein which is very important in the development of fibrous plaque. Second, fish oils reduce plasma fibrinogen concentrations in human subjects. Fibrinogen is essential for clot formation and is a significant risk factor for coronary artery disease. Third, they reduce the viscosity of whole blood, thereby very likely providing better oxygen supply to tissues. Fourth, they increase clot dissolving activity by increasing plasminogen activator. Fifth, they usually reduce blood pressure in both short and long term studies. Sixth, EPA increases the endotheliums ability to relax the coronary arteries.

There are now two controlled studies reporting that fish oils sharply inhibit atherosclerosis in coronary angioplasty (dilating the diseased coronary artery with a balloon cathether) patients. In one study, 82 patients were enrolled. Four months after the procedure, 36% of the control group had renarrowing of their arteries but only 16% of the fish oil group did. There were no side effects from the fish oils.

There is now a great deal of epidemiology supporting the animal and human experiments. A twenty year study in the Netherlands reported a 50% reduction in heart disease death rate for men eating 7 ounces of fish per week. The Western Electric study found lower heart death with more fish. Swedish and Japanese surveys have also found less atherosclerosis in fish eaters.

SUMMARY AND RECOMMENDATIONS: EPA

When comparing the benefits of EPA to linoleic acid, it should be noted it takes 20 to 40 grams of linoleic acid to moderately inhibit platelet aggregation and reduce serum cholesterol. Linoleic acid has an unpredictable effect on triglyceride levels. EPA, in contrast, is effective on a broader spectrum of risk factors with doses of 2 to 10 grams. EPA consistently reduces serum triglyceride, cholesterol, and LDL, while the beneficial HDL is often increased. Platelet aggregation is decreased and bleeding times lengthened. Animal and human work support these findings.

We saw there is a growing body of diverse and powerful evidence supporting fish oils as being protective, from blood pressure to endothelium and atherosclerosis. Certainly the data on fish oils is far more impressive than on any other type of oil, whether it be olive, corn, soybean or other polyunsaturated vegetable oil.

The best sources of EPA are fish oils and fatty fish, such as salmon, mackerel, herring, sardines, albacore tuna and catfish. These fish provide about 4 to 6 grams of EPA per half pound, which is a clinically effective dose. Caution should be exercised with cod liver oil because of potential vitamin D toxicity. Remember, excessive vitamin D is given to animals to promote atherosclerosis. One tablespoon of cod liver oil provides almost 2 grams of EPA but it also supplies an excessive 1200 IU of vitamin D. EPA supplements are available. It would seem prudent not to go beyond 5 grams per day if one chose to supplement, otherwise you are going beyond the average consumption of the Eskimos. A good solution is to include more salmon, catfish, albacore tuna, sardines, mackerel and other fish in your diet.

REFERENCES

GENERAL REVIEW and CRITICAL ARTICLES

Ahrens, E. The diet-heart question in 1985: has it really been settled? Lancet 1:1085-87,1985.

Anderson, K. et. al. Cholesterol & Mortality, 30 year follow up-Framingham Study. JAMA 257:2176-80,1987.

Bonanome, A. & Grundy, S. Effect of stearic acid on plasma cholesterol. N Engl J Med 318:1244-8,1988.

Goodnight, Scott, et.al. Polyunsaturated Fatty Acids, Hyperlipidemia and Thrombosis. Arterio 2:87-113,1982.

Gorringe, Why blame butter? J Roy Soc Med 79:661-3,1986.

Gotto, A. et. al. Hyperlipidemia: A complete approach. Patient Care 23 #3:34-54,1989.

Grundy, Scott, et. al. Rationale of the Diet-Heart Statement of the American Heart Assn. Circ 65:839A-854A,1982

Levy, Robert, Declining Mortality in Coronary Heart Disease Arteriosclerosis 1:312-325,1981

McGill, H. Relationship of Dietary Cholesterol to Serum Cholesterol & to Athero. Am J Clin Nutr 32:2664-2702,1979.

Raymond, C. Dietary cholesterol still a lively discussion topic. JAMA 259:1435-6,1988.

Roberts, L. Measuring cholesterol is as tricky as lowering it. Science 238:482-3,1987.

Stehbens, W. An appraisal of the epidemic rise of coronary heart disease & its decline. Lancet 1:606-10,1987.

OXIDIZED CHOLESTEROL

Anonymous, Atherosclerosis and auto-oxidation of cholesterol Lancet 1:964-965,1980.

Baranowski, A. et.al. Connective tissue responses to oxysterols. Athero 41:255-266,1982

Imai, H. et.al. Angiotoxicity and arteriosclerosis due to oxidized cholesterol. Arch Path Lab Med 100:565-72,1976.

Imai, H. et.al. Angiotoxicity of oxygenated sterols and possible precursors. Science 207:651-653,1980.

Johnson, M. Cholesterol oxides in Indian Ghee. Lancet 2: 656-58, 1987.

Taylor, C. et.al. Spontaneously occuring angiotoxic derivitives of cholesterol. Am J Clin Nutr 32:40-57,1979.

OMEGA-3 FATTY ACIDS

Anonymous, Experimental Myocardial Infarction and Fish Oil Nutrition Reviews 39:316-317,1981

Culp, B.,et. al. The effect of dietary fish oil on experimental MI. Prostaglan 20:1021-31,1980.

Dehmer, G. et.al. Reduction in the rate of retenosis after angioplasty by fish oils. N Eng J Med 319:733-40,1988.

Fox & DiCorleto, Fish oils inhibit endothelial cell production of PDGF like protein. Science 241:453-56,1988.

Goodnight, et. al. PUFA, hyperlipidemia and thrombosis. Arterio 2:87-113,1982.

Hay, C. et.al. Effect of Fish Oil on Platelet Kinetics in Patients With IHD. Lancet 1,1269-72,1982

Hostmark, A. et.al. Fish oil and plasma fibrinogen. Br Med J 297:180-1,1988.

Leaf, A. & Weber, P. Cardiovascular effects of n-3 fatty acids. N Engl J Med 318:549-57,1988.

Saynor,R. and Verel,D. Eicosapentaenoic acid, bleeding time and Serum Lipids. Lancet 2:272,1982

Singer, P. et.al. Long term effect of mackerel on blood pressure, lipids & TXA-2. Athero 62:259-65,1986.

OTHER TOPICS

Antar, M. et.al. Changes in Retail Market Food Supplies in the U.S. in the Last 70 Years in Relation to the Incidence of CHD. Am J Clin Nutr 14:169-78,1961.

Friend, B. Nutrients in United States Food Supply. Am J Clin Nutr 20:907-14,1967

Gordon, T. et.al. Diet and Its Relation to CHD and Death in Three Populations. Circ 63:500-15,1981.

Lipid Research Clinics Program. Lipid research clinics coronary primary prevention trial. JAMA 251:351-64,1983.

Miller, G. & Miller, N. Plasma HDL Conc. and Development of Ischaemic Heart Disease. Lancet 1:16-19,1975

Miller, G. High Density Lipoproteins and Atherosclerosis. Ann Rev Med 31:97-108,1980

Pomrehn, Paul, et. al. Ischemic Heart Disease Mortality in Iowa Farmers. JAMA 248:1073-76,1982

Welsh, S.& Marston, R. Review of Trends in Food in The U.S. 1909-1980. J Am Diet Assn 81:120-5,1982

3. MAGNESIUM and CARDIOVASCULAR DISEASE

There is a surprisingly rich literature on magnesium and cardiovascular disease (CVD). A steady stream of monographs and reviews have documented magnesium's role as an important protective factor. Seelig's 1964 and 1974 reviews along with her remarkable 1980 monograph provides the most thorough and extensive discussion of magnesium and CVD available. Any reader interested in investigating magnesium further would be well advised to begin with Seelig's work. Even though there is a plethora of important material available, the critical role of magnesium in CVD is neglected by many physicians and dietitians. The excessive attention paid to fat, cholesterol, and sodium appears to have crowded magnesium out of the spotlight.

INFARCTS AND ATHEROSCLEROSIS

There are some studies on the effects of pure magnesium deficiency on the arteries of experimental animals. The ones that have been performed on dogs, rats and cows have shown thickened intima, smooth muscle proliferation along with degeneration of elastic fibers, calcification and edema. These changes are similar to the early stages of atherosclerosis in humans, especially in infants and children. Heart muscle necrosis, calcification and fibrosis also occured in animals on magnesium deficient diets.

High calcium and/or high vitamin D diets exacerbate the damage, especially calcification, done by low magnesium diets. Higher intakes of magnesium reversed these effects. Seelig and others have shown high vitamin D and calcium increases the requirement for magnesium and intensifies magnesium deficiencies. It has been known for many years that high vitamin D regimens promote atherosclerosis in animals. Magnesium supplements have prevented many of the effects of high vitamin D diets such as hypertension, calcification and hypercholesterolemia.

High fat diets (combined with excessive vitamin D, casein, sugar and thyroid gland removal) have tradionally been used to produce vascular pathology in animals. A number of investigators report magnesium rich regimens protect against and low magnesium diets intensify the damage done by high fat diets. The amount of fat and cholesterol deposited in the arteries was decreased with magnesium supplements. Raised intimal plaques, elastic degeneration and calcification occuring in fat fed rabbits were prevented with magnesium supplements. In all animals species studied, magnesium supplements protect against fat promoted arterial pathology.

A visciously pathological diet producing myocardial infarcts in 80 to 90% of the animals subjected to it has been developed by several researchers. In addition to the high myocardial infarct rate, these regimens produced extensive atherosclerosis, calcification and increased blood coagulation. The pathological diet, often dubed the cardiovasopathic diet, is low in magnesium, potassium and chloride but rich in saturated fat, cholesterol, protein, vitamin D, sodium and phosphate. This regimen is not dissimilar to many American diets except for the low chloride. Restoring normal intakes of salts including magnesium reduced the incidence of myocardial infarct from 90% to 13% even though saturated fat, cholesterol, protein and vitamin D remained high. When animals were put on the pathological diet but given five times the normal magnesium chloride there was a striking reduction in myocardial infarcts and atherosclerosis. These experiments which were done on cocks, rats and dogs support magnesium as an extremely important factor for preventing heart disease.

MAGNESIUM and STRESS

Magnesium, stress and cardiovascular disease has been extensively studied in animals. Many experiments have clearly demonstrated higher rates of cardiac damage in stressed, magnesium deficient animals than in stressed magnesium sufficient animals. Adrenalin, one of the hormones released during stress, depletes heart and blood vessel magnesium. Adrenalin infusion produces arterial lesions. They are similar to lesions produced by pure magnesium deficiency, suggesting adrenalin's induction of cellular magnesium deficiency may be the mechanism of arterial damage by adrenalin.

Recently, Classen investigated the effects of adrenalin on magnesium deficient animals. Seventy two percent of the magnesium deprived animals developed large heart necroses compared to none in the magnesium adequate controls. Interestingly, serum magnesium levels rose in the magnesium deficient animals after adrenalin administration, emphasizing the unreliability of serum magnesium as a measure of tissue status. Classen demonstrated magnesium supplements protected magnesium deficient animals against adrenalin's damage.

In another set of experiments, magnesium deficient rats were pretreated with stress hormones (9-fluorocortisol and adrenalin). Animals not supplemented with magnesium developed cardiac hypertrophy and an extremely high incidence (83%) of cardiac necrosis. There were a variety of magnesium supplements used. All of them prevented the cardiac hypertrophy but some of the supplements only moderately reduced the incidence and severity of cardiac necroses. Surprisingly, only the magnesium supplements containing chloride (such as magnesium chloride or magnesium aspartate hydrochloride) significantly reduced the incidence and severity of the cardiac necroses.

HYPOXIA and ARRHYTHMIA: ANIMAL WORK

Cardiac and vascular smooth muscle have greatly increased tendencies for contraction when there is lack of oxygen in the tissues (hypoxia). Experimental animals with ligated coronary arteries readily develop arrhythmia and ventricular fibrillation. Vascular smooth muscle spasms are produced more easily under hypoxic conditions. Intravenous magnesium sulfate and to a greater extent magnesium chloride suppressed arrhythmias in dogs with constricted coronary arteries. In another set of experiments magnesium protected against hypoxia induced ventricular fibrillation in dogs. Infusions of mineral solutions without magnesium did not retard the ventricular fibrillations. Hypoxia experiments on pigs, rats and rabbits have shown magnesium infusions to be protective. In rats made hypoxic, pretreatment with magnesium chloride for five days also prevented cardiac necroses.

Many of the studies show parallel and synergistic protective effects when potassium is administered alone or in combination with magnesium. This is reasonable since magnesium deficiency results in cellular losses of potassium. The potassium uptake by cells is restricted when there is concurrent magnesium deficiency. Magnesium is needed by the enzyme ATPase, which is essential for pumping potassium into cells and sodium out of cells. Potassium deficient cells are not benefited by potassium supplements if simultaneous magnesium deficiency is present.

In guinea pigs, magnesium and/or potassium aspartates (but not chlorides) protected against ECG changes and tachycardia induced by hypoxia. In additional experiments, magnesium aspartates doubled the tolerance for hypoxia in guinea pigs. Other studies on rats, rabbits and guinea pigs have shown similar protective effects for magnesium and potassium aspartates but not for the chlorides.

Magnesium deficiencies, per se, in animals without hypoxia or other stresses produce serious arrhythmias and abnormal ECG's. These effects have been documented in dogs, rabbits, rats, cows, pigs, and guinea pigs. Seelig has pointed out that "the ECG of magnesium deficiency also resembles that seen in myocardial ischemia of coronary insufficiency: flattened, inverted or peaked T waves and ST depression, as well as abnormally long QT interval. It's ST depression and T wave inversion also resemble the ECG of subendocardial infarction." (Seelig, 1980, pg 222)

An important investigation of magnesium and the electrical stability of dogs hearts was reported by Ghani and Rabah. Hearts of intact dogs, dogs given digitalis (digitalis increases the incidence of arrhythmias and magnesium protects against digitalis induced arrhythmias), and denervated heart-lung preparations were electrically stimulated to determine their ventricular premature contraction threshold and ventricular fibrillation threshold. After magnesium chloride infusion, the thresholds for ventricular premature contractions increased significantly. After magnesium administration, the thresholds for ventricular fibrillation tripled in intact animals, doubled in intact digitalized dogs and heart lung preparations. These experiments provide powerful support that magnesium protects against arrhythmia and fibrillation.

In other experiments on rat hearts, Hearse et. al. reported magnesium was the most effective agent they have tested for protection against ischemia. In their 1978 publication they determined the optimum concentration of magnesium for ischemic protection.

HUMAN WORK

Human work has convincingly supported magnesium's role in the electrical stability of the heart. Davis and Ziady gave 240 to 360 mg of magnesium (in the form of 2 to 3 grams of magnesium chloride hexahydrate) for 2 years to 25 patients with ECG abnormalities. They found a pronounced decrease in the QT and QU intervals. Increased QT intervals are strongly associated with sudden heart death. The normalization of QT intervals in this study is a significant finding.

Experimental magnesium deficiency in human subjects produced similar ECG abnormalities including increased QT intervals. Magnesium repletion of these subjects normalized their ECG's.

Open heart surgery causes significant heart muscle magnesium losses. Scheinman et. al. in 1969 stopped fibrillation in several open heart surgery patients using intravenous magnesium. Buky in 1970 spontaneously stopped fibrillation in eighteen open heart surgery patients with intravenous magnesium. Holden in 1978 did a controlled trial on 70 heart surgery patients. The patients given magnesium sulfate post operatively had fewer postoperative problems and a much lower rate of atrial fibrillation (1 vs 12). He also reported on another set of 11 heart surgery patients who had ventricular fibrillations which did not respond to standard therapy. When these patients were administered intravenous magnesium, their ventricular fibrillations stopped within two minutes.

Magnesium infusions were first shown to protect against digitalis arrhythmias in humans in 1935. Many clinical reports since then have confirmed magnesium's beneficial effect on digitalis toxicity. Animal experiments also have confirmed the anti-arrhythmic effect.

Cohen and Kitzes recently reported their clinical experience with seven congestive heart disease patients with digitalis-toxic arrhythmias. They gave them intravenous and intramuscular magnesium producing almost immediate normalization of their heart rhythms. It is instructive to note five of the seven patients had normal serum magnesium levels. This finding reconfirms the many previous papers claiming serum magnesium concentrations are not reliable indicators of cellular magnesium status. Red blood cell and lymphocyte magnesium concentrations have been used with some success to evaluate status.

Tissue concentrations of magnesium are ten times greater than serum concentrations and they are often not in equilibrium with each other. Infarcted, ischemic or damaged tissue normally releases magnesium into the serum, resulting in elevation of serum magnesium levels. We have the paradox, that just at the time when tissue concentrations are at their lowest, the serum concentrations are raised. This is one of the reasons the measurement of serum magnesium is not a reliable indicator of tissue status. The lack of reliability is a major reason magnesium is relatively neglected by many cardiologists.

Iseri et. al. in 1975 reported serious ventricular arrhythmias in two magnesium depleted alcoholics responded rapidly to magnesium infusions. The arrhythmias had been resistant to standard therapy before magnesium administration Magnesium deficiency is common in alcoholics due to poor diets and higher magnesium excretion rates. Paradoxically, cessation of alcohol drinking often results in a rapid fall in serum magnesium. Many hospitals routinely supplement alcoholics with magnesium to prevent convulsions.

In 1983, Iseri et. al. sucessfully treated 3 patients who had normal serum magnesium and episodes of intractable ventricular tachycardia and ventricular fibrillation. These patients did not respond to standard strategies for arrhythmias, but dramatically improved with magnesium infusions. These patients illustrate the well established fact that normal magnesium levels can exist with concurrent cellular magnesium deficiency.

Clinical reports of magnesium usage during myocardial ischemia have shown striking benefit. Angina patients given magnesium intramuscularly by Malkiel-Shapiro responded with decreased pain and reduced nitroglycerine usage. In another trial of 64 acute myocardial infarct patients, intramuscular magnesium sharply reduced mortality in the group. Parsons, in a series of 33 myocardial infarct patients claimed magnesium reduced mortality, decreased angina and improved their ECG's. Melon, using magnesium and potassium aspartates reported greatly improved ECG's in myocardial infarct patients. Several other researchers report magnesium and potassium aspartates plus glucose (and insulin in some cases) rapidly reduces angina pain. Seelig cites a number of other papers documenting the beneficial effect of magnesium in acute ischemic heart disease.

Recently a number of clinicians have found benefit using magnesium salts on patients. Cohen and Kitzes in 1984 used iv magnesium sulfate to terminate 41 episodes of resting angina in fifteen patients. In four out of four patients magnesium therapy prevented further attacks. Morton et. al. in 1984 reduced infarct size in a group of patients compared to controls using iv magnesium sulfate. There was also a remarkable decrease in ventricular premature beats and lidocaine usage in the magnesium group. Perticone used magnesium sulfate to stop dangerous ventricular arrhythmias in 10 patients.

In the largest double blind study done to date, Rasmussen et. al. reported a sharp drop in mortality (7% vs 19% for controls) during the first four weeks in myocardial infarct patients receiving iv magnesium chloride. Also, 47% of the placebo group had arrhythmias needing treatment compared to only 21% of the magnesium group. There were no adverse effects of the iv magnesium therapy observed.

POTASSIUM AND MAGNESIUM

Animal and human work demonstrate magnesium deficiency can lead to intercellular potassium deficits. The explanation given for this phenomenon is the enzyme (sodium potassium ATPase) which pumps potassium across cell membranes into the cell requires magnesium, hence magnesium deficiency results in less potassium pumped into cells.

It is well known that most diuretics increase potassium excretion but less generally known that they increase magnesium excretion also. It is not uncommon for long term diuretic patients to become refractive to potassium repletion therapy. There are several reports demonstrating cellular potassium repletion is impeded because of a concurrent magnesium deficiency. For example, Dyckner and Wester in 1978 studied 50 long term diuretic patients who had frequent ventricular extrasystoles. Potassium supplements did not reduce the extrasystoles or replenish the depleted intracellular potassium. In contrast, infusion of magnesium significantly increased intercellular potassium and markedly reduced the frequency of arrhythmias.

Dyckner and Wester also investigated 8 patients suffering from diuretic induced low serum sodium levels and concurrent high intercellular sodium levels. Paradoxically, increased intake of sodium aggravates the condition and can lead to death. In these patients, magnesium infusion normalized serum sodium, lowered intercellular sodium and raised intercellular potassium. All of these effects were extremely beneficial for the patients. In a separate study, these investigators gave 20 hypertensives, who were on long term diuretic therapy, magnesium supplements (365 mg of magnesium in the form of 3690 mg of magnesium aspartate hydrochloride). After six months there was an average reduction in systolic and diastolic pressure of 12 and 8 mmHg respectively.

It appears magnesium supplements are beneficial for diuretic patients. Magnesium reduces the arrhythmias, improves potassium and sodium concentrations and reduces blood pressure.

MAGNESIUM AND SERUM LIPIDS

There are several reasons why magnesium is relatively neglected by cardiologists. First and probably most important is the unreliability and unpredictabiltiy of serum magnesium as a measurement of magnesium status. Several studies, for example, have shown elevated serum magnesium after an MI, whereas others have reported depressed serum magnesium. Since infarcted, and to a lesser extent ischemic, tissue loses magnesium to the serum, normal or elevated serum magnesium levels can mask a deficient tissue concentration and can be a symptom of recently infarcted or ischemic tissue.

Another major reason for magnesium's neglect is the confusing and unpredictable effect magnesium has on blood lipids. Traditionally, any substance or agent which lowers serum cholesterol or triglyceride receives immediate attention by the scientific establishment and the public. Anything which does not lower serum lipids is often ignored for possible utility in CVD (unless it is a patentable item such as a beta blocker or calcium antagonist).

When looking at serum lipids and serum magnesium in humans, a consistent relationship has never been found. This suggests serum lipids and serum magnesium do not influence each other. It also likely means they are affected by different dietary factors.

Giving magnesium supplements to humans does not influence serum lipids predictably. Intramuscular administration appears to mildly lower serum cholesterol, but this is an impractical means to lower serum cholesterol. Animal experiments are inconsistent in their results. Some report raised serum lipids with magnesium supplements, some report no effect and others show a drop in serum lipids. This supports our general conclusion that magnesium does not affect serum lipids to any great degree.

There is limited evidence from human and animal work suggesting that high fat intake impairs magnesium absorption. Unfortunately the human trials were for ten days or less. There has been sparce animal work, but the little done has demonstrated high fat diets inhibit magnesium absorption.

EPIDEMIOLOGY AND TISSUE LEVELS

Chipperfield and Chipperfield compared heart muscle magnesium levels in 81 persons dying of heart disease and 158

non-heart disease controls.   Those dying of sudden heart
death had 17% less heart muscle magnesium than controls and
46% higher heart calcium levels.   Magnesium is a calcium
antagonist, so the low concentration of magnesium in the
heart muscle could account for the elevated calcium concentrations.   Both low magnesium and high calcium increase the
heart muscles irritability and tendency for arrhythmia.   The
non-sudden heart death group had 7% lower magnesium and 10%
higher calcium levels.   Elwood et. al. in the largest autopsy
study done on magnesium, comprising 1236 samples, found a 12%
lower magnesium concentration in sudden heart death and a 17%
lower concentration in non-sudden heart death.   Several other
investigators have confirmed the finding of lower heart
magnesium concentrations in persons dying of ischemic heart
disease.

Statistics on water hardness, both nationally and internationally , generally show hard water areas have lower heart
disease death rates than soft water areas.   Both higher
magnesium and calcium content of water correlates with lower
death rates.   Some statistical analyses of the hard water
data report a better protective effect for magnesium than for
calcium.   This type of evidence can not be used as proof for
magnesium's role as a protective factor, but along with the
animal, cellular and human work, it does provide another
important piece of data supporting magnesium's protective
role.

Anderson's autopsy work suggests the magnesium content
of the heart muscle is related to the magnesium content of
the water in the area.   He finds higher heart muscle magnesium in hard water areas when comparing non-heart attack and
heart attack deaths in different areas.   He has also found in
the populations he has studied, the major difference between
hard and soft water death rates is the higher sudden heart
death rate in soft water areas.   This is consistent with the
animal and human work on magnesium and fibrillation.
Ventricular fibrillation is a major cause of sudden heart
death.

In Finland the magnesium content of soil appears to be an
important risk factor.   In northeastern Finland, the heart
death rate is twice that of southwestern Finland.   Northeastern Finland has one of the highest heart death rates in
the world.   The soil magnesium content in northeastern

Finland is one third that of southwestern Finland, providing another piece of support for the magnesium hypothesis.

STATUS

Serum magnesium does not correlate with total body magnesium, nevertheless status is usually evaluated in serum, a far from ideal location for magnesium assessment. Accepted serum values for normal status are 0.7 to 1.0 mmole/L (1.4 to 2 meq/L or 1.7 to 2.4 mg/dL) but it is well established that a normal serum level can mask a deficient tissue level. Dorup et. al., for example, in 1988 found 15 out of 25 diuretic patients with normal serum magnesium but deficient tissue content of magnesium.

For readers interested in extensive discussion of tests for magnesium deficiency, you should consult the appendix of Seelig's 1980 monograph. She reviews the following sites and methods for determining magnesium status: serum; erythrocyte; skeletal muscle; white blood cell; and percentage retention of parenteral magnesium loads. The monograph contains a vast bibliography, over 2,000 references from the scientific literature on magnesium.

CLINICAL CONDITIONS AFFECTING MAGNESIUM STATUS

A number of conditions are associated with magnesium depletion. Extended fasting for two months or longer can produce marked loss of magnesium. Prolonged vomiting results in significant magnesium loss. Many chronic gastrointestinal disorders such as malabsorption, enteritis, celiac disease, ulcerative colitis and acute pancreatitis often have concurrent hypomagnesia. Burn victims, diabetics, patients with renal disease, preeclampsia and eclampsia are all conditions strongly associated with magnesium deficiencies.

Alcoholism is invariably linked with poor magnesium status. Serum levels are usually lower but the more reliable red blood cell concentration is always low in alcoholics with delirium tremens. A rapid fall in serum magnesium often occurs when drinking ceases. The rapid fall takes place at the same time convulsions begin.

Patients on thiazide or loop diuretics are at risk of developing magnesium or potassium deficiencies. Also, Whang recently showed a high percentage of poor magnesium status in patients receiving digitalis. Many, but not all of these patients were on diuretics.

DIETARY FACTORS AND MAGNESIUM

Calcium and magnesium have many interdependent relationships. Long term magnesium deficits in human and animals (except the rat) produce depressed serum calcium values which are not improved with calcium supplements. Calcification of soft tissue, such as, heart, artery, muscles, kidney, and joints is a routine finding in magnesium deficient animals. It would seem reasonable to expect this in humans also. Membrane and tissue studies have shown magnesium is a calcium antagonist (ie. inhibits the influx of calcium into cells), hence calcium accumulates in magnesium deficient cells. Human and animal work has demonstrated high cell calcium occurs with magnesium deficiency.

The finding of high cell calcium with low magnesium is probably an important factor in muscular hyperexcitability, arrhythmias and convulsions. All three of these conditions are exhibited in animals (and very probably in humans) when they are made magnesium deficient.

Magnesium deficient muscle cells require less voltage for a contraction, hence they have a greater tendency for contraction, spasm or convulsion. A high influx of calcium into muscle cells increases muscle contraction, so low magnesium plus high calcium influx is a very good combination for producing hyperexcitable muscles, arrhythmias and convulsions.

There is good animal evidence to show the cellular accumulation of calcium is independent of dietary calcium. Alcoholics are good examples of this. They have notoriously low intakes of almost all nutrients including calcium and magnesium, but they exhibit strikingly elevated cell calcium concentrations. Their low intake of magnesium is likely an important factor in their cellular accumulation of calcium.

High dietary intakes of calcium impair magnesium absorption and exacerbates magnesium deficiencies in animals.

Human work has demonstrated this effect also. Persons with high consumption of calcium (above 1300 mg) or who supplement with substantial amounts of calcium run the risk of gradual magnesium depletion unless extra dietary or supplemental magnesium is provided (daily intake should be above 400 mg).

Vitamin D is usually added to milk and calcium supplements to increase calcium absorption. Very high doses of vitamin D given in animal and human experiments, indicates excessive vitamin D moderately impairs magnesium absorption. The RDA for vitamin D is 200 IU for adults, but several surveys have reported many people consume more than 1200 IU per day, primarily from excessive supplementation. Since vitamin D is a steroid, which moderately impairs magnesium status and promotes, at high doses, atherosclerosis in animals, it seems unwise to supplement with large amounts. Almost all multivitamin supplements contain 400 IU of vitamin D, so persons taking many different supplements every day run the risk of overdosing with vitamin D unless they carefully read labels.(see Chapter 8).

Diets with excessive phosphates raise the magnesium requirement. Phosphates inhibit magnesium absorption and increase magnesium excretion in animals. Phosphates added to atherogenic diets increase the incidence and severity of cardiovascular pathology in experimental animals. In the United States many people ingest considerably more than the RDA (800 mg) of phosphate because of our high protein and soda pop consumption. Many soft drinks are formulated with phosphates. One 12 ounce bottle of cola can contain up to 400 mg of phosphate. Persons who drink excessive soft drinks should check the labels in order to select types which do not contain phosphates. There is evidence phosphate consumption has gone up sharply since the early 1900's, mainly due to our love of soft drinks.

Concerning fats, we have previously pointed out dietary fat moderately inhibits magnesium absorption. Magnesium requirements are raised somewhat on high fat diets. In the U.S. 38% of our calories come from fat, a factor which increases our magnesium requirements.

Phytates inhibit the absorption of magnesium, calcium, iron and zinc by forming insoluble compounds with these nutrients. Phytates are found primarily in the bran of various grains such as wheat, rice, oats and soybeans. Whole wheat flour and brown rice contain more phytates than refined flour or polished rice. Short term experiments on humans in which whole wheat or brown rice is introduced show significantly decreased magnesium absorption even though whole wheat and other whole grain products contain much more magnesium than polished grain products (145 mg/100g for whole wheat vs 40 mg/100g for white flour).

Most studies demonstrate after several weeks on high phytate regimens, magnesium absorption steadily increases to its former value. This suggests our digestive tracts can adjust to a high phytate diet. Most of the studies used unleavened bread which inhibits magnesium much more than leavened bread. The yeast in leavened bread alters the phytates so they do not interfere with absorption as much.

Several tentative conclusions can be made on phytates: 1. Phytates increase magnesium requirements. 2. Foods with phytates are usually high in magnesium. 3. Over a period of time, digestive tracts adjust to high phytate diets with increased magnesium absorption. 4. Magnesium is better absorbed from whole grain breads than whole grain crackers or other unleavened whole grain products.

The results on protein's effect on magnesium is confusing. Very low protein intake, at least in the few studies reported, appears to decrease magnesium status. Increasing the protein moderately improves magnesium status, but when excessive protein is given, magnesium excretion increases considerably. In the U.S. many people have excessive intakes of protein. The limited experiments would suggest our high protein intakes are increasing our magnesium requirements. Animal studies support this conclusion.

MAGNESIUM REQUIREMENTS

The National Research Council in 1980 set the recommended dietary allowance (RDA) for magnesium at 300 mg for a 132 pound female and 350 mg for a 154 pound male. They recommend 150 mg more during pregnancy and lactation. (See Seelig 1980 for the critical importance of adequate magnesium during pregnancy and lactation.)

Seelig (1964,1980,and 1981) has exhaustively reviewed the literature and concluded the 300 and 350 mg figures should be increased for the recommended allowances. Seelig's detailed examination of magnesium balance studies reveals most of the experiments did not consider sweat losses. When sweat is accounted for, many more subjects would be in negative balance at 300 and 350 mg. Analysis of balance studies suggests it takes 450 mg for females and 500 mg for males to have 90% of the subjects in balance.

Magnesium is carefully conserved by the kidney during periods of low intake. This fact could make balance studies invalid for determining magnesium requirements. The body could reestablish equilibrium between input and output of magnesium at low intake even though tissue levels were not at optimum concentrations. Indeed, early work demonstrates balance can be established at suboptimum intakes. One study showed subjects in balance with 350 mg of magnesium per day (the RDA) for 8 weeks, and then given magnesium supplements had large retention of magnesium (2000 to 3000 mg per week). The retention with supplements indicates the previous 8 weeks on RDA amounts of magnesium was not adequate. A 44 week study of healthy college men showed marked retention during most periods on 600 mg magnesium. Other reports have confirmed RDA amounts are not adequate for many subjects and should be raised to 450 and 500 mg for females and males respectively.

Another problem with the balance studies used to establish the RDA is they do not incorporate factors found in the typical American diet which raise magnesium requirements, such as high calcium, phosphate, vitamin D and protein. One sixty day balance study done on 15 young women consuming 285 mg of magnesium did include extra calcium and phosphate. The women were in strong negative balance (they were losing 50 mg per day) because of high calcium (1040 mg) and high phosphate (1550 mg) ingestion. In addition to dietary factors, stress increases magnesium requirements. The effects of stress have not been in the RDA calculations. These are some of the reasons why it may be prudent to raise the RDA to 500 mg for males and 450 for females.

It is almost academic to discuss raising the RDA because most Americans do not consume 300 to 350 mg per day. Many dietary surveys report daily intakes ranging from 150 to 300 mg. A recent survey of diets in 50 colleges showed an average magnesium content of 250 mg, but calcium and phosphorous were 1200 mg and 1700 mg, respectively. The high values for calcium and phosphorous put greater stress on magnesium status.

Analysis of Oriental diets have shown different patterns. Usually magnesium is above 450 mg but calcium and phosphorous are below 700 mg. These numbers are favorable for good magnesium status. Possibly this is one of the reasons for the low rate of coronary artery disease in the Orient.

The reasons for our low magnesium diets are straight forward. Our meals average 38% fat, 14% sugar and 20% polished grains. Fat and sugar contain no magnesium and polished grains have about 70% of their magnesium striped out when they are refined.

The best sources of magnesium are green leafy vegetables, whole grains, beans, nuts, seeds, seafoods and some vegetables. Three ounce servings of these foods provide the following amounts of magnesium: whole wheat flour 140 mg, white flour 35 mg, whole barley 160 mg, oats 115 mg, brown rice 95mg, white rice 25 mg, nuts 120 to 250 mg, shell fish 40 to 120 mg, dried legumes 120 to 250 mg, green leafy vegetables 50 to 100 mg, fish 20 to 50 mg, corn 35 mg, banana 35 mg, potato 25 mg, celery 25 mg, and meats 15 to 25 mg.

SUMMARY and RECOMMENDATIONS

There is an extensive and impressive body of evidence supporting magnesium as a protective factor against hypoxia, atherosclerosis, arrhythmia and infarct. Magnesium deficiencies are associated with higher rates of arrhythmia, infarct and atherosclerosis. Diets rich in fat, sugar, and polished grains will be poor in magnesium. The work on magnesium makes a persuasive case for having diets rich in whole grains, legumes, green leafy vegetables, nuts and seeds (in limited amounts) and low in fat, sugar, and polished grains.

Persons with low magnesium diets would be wise to change their diet or to supplement. Magnesium oxide, magnesium hydroxide and magnesium carbonate are common supplements. If supplementing, 200 mg per day is a reasonable and safe amount. There is a wide margin of safety for magnesium, but excessive supplementation with a mineral normally impairs the absorption of some other mineral.

REFERENCES

Anonymous, Magnesium Deficiency and Ischemic Heart Disease Nutr Rev 46:311-312,1988

Burch, G. & Giles, T., The Importance of Magnesium Deficiency in Cardiovascular Disease. Am Heart J 94:649-57,1977

Chadda,K. et.al. Magnesium and Cardiac Arrhythmia in Patients With Acute Infarction-Preliminary Observations in Magnesium in Health and Disease. Cantin & Seelig,eds. 1980, pp 545-549.

Chipperfield & Chipperfield, Metal Content of Heart Muscle in Death from IHD. Am Heart J 95:732-7,1978.

Chipperfield and Chipperfield, Magnesium and the Heart. Am Heart J 93:679-82,1977.

Classen, H., Magnesium and Cardiac Necroses. J Internat Acad Prev Med 6:119-37,1980.

Cohen, L. and Kitzes, R., Magnesium Sulfate and Digitalis Toxic Arrhythmias. JAMA 249:2808-10,1983.

Cohen & Kitzes, Magnesium sulfate in the Treatment of Variant Angina. Magnesium 3:46-49,1984

Davis, W.& Ziady, F. Effect of Oral Magnesium Chloride on the QTc and QUc Intervals of the EKG. SA Med J 53:591-3,1978.

Dorup, I. et. al. Reduced conc. of K, Mg and Na-K pumps in skeletal muscle using diuretics. Br Med J 296:455-8,1988

Dyckner, T. and Wester, P. Intracellular Potassium After Magnesium Infusion. Brit Med J 1:822-3,1978

Dyckner, T. and Wester, P. Effects of Magnesium Infusions in Diuretic Induced Hyponatraemia. Lancet 1:585-6,1981.

Dyckner, T and Wester, P. Effect of Magnesium on Blood Pressure. Brit Med J 286:1847-9,1983.

Elwood, P. and Beasley, W. Myocardial Magnesium and Ischaemic Heart Disease. Artery 9:200-4,1981.

Ghani, M. and Rabah, M. Effect of Magnesium Chloride on Electrical Stability of the Heart. Am Heart J 94:600-2,1977.

Hearse, D. et.al. Myocardial Protection During Ischemic Cardiac Arrest- The Importance of Magnesium in Cardioplegic Infusates. J Thoracic CV Surg 75:877-85,1978.

Iseri, L. et.al. Magnesium Deficiency and Cardiac Disorders Am J Med 58:837-45,1975.

Iseri,L. et.al. Magnesium therapy for Intractable Ventricular Tachyarrhythmias in Normomagnesemic Patients. Western J Med 138:823-8,1983.

Karppanen, H. Epidemiological Studies on the Relationship Between Magnesium Intake & CVD. Artery 9:190-9,1981.

Linden, V. Correlation of Vitamin D Intake to Ischemic Heart Disease, Hypercholesterolemia, and Renal Calcinosis. in Nutritional Imbalances in Infant and Adult Disease. Seelig, ed. 1977, pp 23-42.

Masironi, R. & Shaper, A. Epidem. Studies of Health Effects of Water From Different Sources. Ann Rev Nutr 1:375-400,1981

Mather, W. et.al. Hypomagnesaemia in Diabetes. Clinica Chimica Acta 95:235-42,1979.

Morton, B. et. al. Magnesium therapy in acute myocardial infarction: a double blind study. Magnesium 3:346-52, 1984

Perticone, F. et.al. Therapeutic use of magnesium sulphate in ventricular arrhythmias. J Am Col Nutr 4:383, 1985 (abstr)

Rasmussen, H. et. al. IV magnesium in acute myocardial infarction. Lancet 1:234-6, 1986.

Seelig, M. The Requirement of Magnesium by the Normal Adult. Am J Clin Nutr 14:342-89,1964.

Seelig, M. and Heggtveit, A. Magnesium Interrelationships in Ischemic Heart Disease Am J Clin Nutr 27:59-79,1974.

Seelig,M. Magnesium Deficiency in The Pathogenesis of Disease Plenum Publishing. New York. 1980

Seelig, M. Magnesium Requirements in Human Nutrition. Magnesium Bulletin 3 (Suppl 1a) 26-47,1981.

Shattock, M. et al. Ionic basis of the Anti-ischemic & anti-arrhythmic properties of Mg.   J Am Col Nutr 6:27-33,1987

Singh, R. et.al. Magnesium in Atherosclerotic Cardiovascular Disease and Sudden Death. Acta Cardiologica 36:411-29,1981.

Turlapaty, P. and Altura, B. Magnesium Deficiency Produces Spasms of Coronary Arteries.   Science 208:198-200,1980.

Weaver, K. Magnesium & its role in vascular reactivity and coagulation.   Contemp Nutr 12 #3, 1987.

Wester, P. Magnesium. Am J Clin Nutr 45:1305-12, 1987.

Whang, R. et. al. Frequency of hypomagnesemia in hospitalized patients receiving digitalis.   Arch Int Med 145:655-6, 1985.

4. COPPER and ZINC

EXCESS COPPER

An influential review published in 1969 titled Trace Elements and Cardiovascular Diseases by Roberto Masironi of the World Health Organization summarized evidence suggesting copper is a promoter of atherosclerosis and CVD. This conclusion was based on three findings. First, giving rabbits excess copper along with high cholesterol diets appeared to increase atherosclerosis. These experiments, published in 1963 to 1966 were flawed because of the extremely high copper doses of 30 to 60 mg which is equivalent to 900 to 1800 mg for a human adult. Since the RDA for humans is 2-3mg, it is doubtful these experiments have any meaning for humans. There have never been any other studies claiming copper promotes atherosclerosis.

Second, a study of males with a history of myocardial infarct (MI) reported higher serum copper in MI patients than in age matched controls. This finding is not a reason for assuming copper causes CVD, since serum copper is controlled by the liver and is relatively independent of diet.

Third, soft water usually contains more copper than hard water because soft water leaches copper out of copper pipes. Soft water is an environmental risk factor for CVD, the softer the water, in general, the higher the death rate. Possibly, but very unlikely, the copper in the soft water was causing the problem. This is the only finding that supports copper as a cause of CVD, but it is very weak evidence. Masironi's most recent review of hard and soft water in the 1981 Annual Reviews of Nutrition did not mention copper as a risk factor in soft water. Frankly, there is meager evidence demonstrating excess copper in our diets causes CVD.

COPPER DEFICIENCY

A recent study by Klevay et. al. provides good evidence that meals low in copper are common in the U.S. The RDA for copper is 2 to 3 mg per day but he found average hospital diets provided 0.76 mg per day. Since the foods analysed in his study are common American foods, it is reasonable to assume people outside hospitals have similar intakes. In fact, Klevay cites 15 other studies on dietary copper, only two were above 2 mg per day and eleven were between 0.2 mg and 1.33 mg per day. A reasonable conclusion from Klevay's work is copper poor diets are quite common and high copper intake is infrequent. Hence the reports claiming excessive copper promotes atherosclerosis in rabbits certainly does not apply to U.S. dietaries. The dietary surveys suggest the opposite question should be asked, that is, do copper deficiencies promote CVD?

Klevay has been a pioneer in providing evidence that copper deficiencies are related to and possibly cause CVD. He formally states his hypothesis as the Zinc/Copper hypothesis of CVD, meaning high intakes of zinc coupled with low amounts of copper promotes CVD. He includes zinc because high zinc exacerbates copper deficiency by inhibiting copper absorption. Nevertheless, except for persons supplementing with large amounts of zinc, diets with excessive zinc are uncommon in the U.S. In this section let's concentrate on the effects of copper deficiencies various researchers have found and look at zinc in the next section.

Hypercholesterolemia, due to higher cholesterol synthesis, can be produced in rats by copper deficient regimens. There is also a decreased percentage of the protective HDL. Two other serum risk factors elevated in low copper rats are uric acid and increased clotting tendency. The Framingham study reported high serum uric acid is associated with higher CVD death rate in humans. The danger of thromboembolism due to increased clotting tendency is self evident. In addition, impaired glucose tolerance, a common risk factor in the U.S., was recently reported to be elevated in copper deficient rats. Serum levels of glucose were increased and insulin release was decreased.

In addition to altered serum factors, there is extensive heart and vascular abnormalities in copper deficient animals. This is not surprising since copper is needed for the synthesis and crosslinking of elastin, an important connective tissue in lung, heart and vascular tissue. Copper deficiency in chickens, pigs and guinea pigs results in decreased elastin content of the blood vessels and eventual aneurysm and rupture of the aorta. Copper poor pigs have died from cardiac failure due to enlarged heart and weakened myocardium. Chickens given reduced copper diets had disrupted elastin, greatly thickened aortic walls and commonly died from internal and subcutaneous hemorrhage. The high incidence of hemorrhage was due to defective elastic tissue in the blood vessels. A more recent study on copper deprived rats produced enlarged, inflamed and hemorrhaging hearts with defective elastic tissue and depleted elastic fibers. In addition, cardiac failure or "falling disease" is found in cattle in Australia grazing on copper depleted soils which can be prevented by the addition of copper to the pasture.

A further finding in rats is electrocardiogram abnormalities similar to those found in high risk humans, such as tall R waves, ST depression, bundle branch block and Q waves. On the other hand, the production of atherosclerotic plaque, the most ubiquitous finding in human CVD, is noticibly absent in copper deficient animals. To date, fibrous plaque has not been produced in animals via copper deprivation.

Little experimental work with copper has been done on humans. Certainly elevated serum glucose, cholesterol and uric acid levels are important risk factors as are abnormal electrocardiograms, depleted and degenerated heart and vessel elastin and increased clotting tendency. Whether these conditions are caused by copper deficiencies in humans remains to be seen. Three pieces of evidence do implicate copper deficiency in human CVD: 1. Persons dying from myocardial infarction have significantly lower heart muscle copper than accident victims. 2. Low to extremely low intakes of copper are common in the U.S. 3. Countries with high intakes of copper have low incidence of CVD. This is not a powerful piece of evidence since countries low in fat, sugar and polished grains are the same countries that are high in copper. Copper primarily occurs in whole grains, legumes and foods low in fat and sugar.

The case for copper is weakened by the paucity of human and primate experimentation. Certainly primates are more appropriate animals for experimentation than rats. In addition, there are three facts on humans which do not fit the copper hypothesis. First, the hard water, soft water data cannot be explained if copper is an important protective agent. Soft water contains more copper, so why are there more CVD deaths in soft water areas? Second, vitamin C supplements in both animals and man impairs copper status, but these same vitamin C supplements lower serum cholesterol in both humans and animals. The copper hypothesis would predict the opposite. Third, large zinc supplements in peripheral vascular disease patients improves the outcome of that disease. These results also contradict Klevay's copper hypothesis.

In 1987 Klevay wrote a review titled "Dietary Copper: A Powerful Determinant of Cholesterolemia" asserting copper is "approximately one hundred times as active in lowering cholesterol in plasma than is clofibrate" (clofibrate is an FDA approved drug to lower serum cholesterol). This sounds exciting and impressive, but Klevay's assertion was based on the results of one experimental subject! Reiser et. al. appeared to support Klevays paper with their report on coppers effect on blood lipoprotein and cholesterol in 24 men. At first reading it looked like copper supplements significantly lowered serum cholesterol and raised HDL after the subjects had been on low copper diets for eleven weeks. The experimental section gave the details of the copper supplement. The supplement was actually Centrum, a popular multivitamin-mineral supplement containing 27 different vitamins and minerals including 3 milligrams of copper. A more accurate statement of Reiser's results would be, 'serum cholesterol is lowered by Centrum in subjects who had previously been on a low copper regimen.

SUMMARY AND RECOMMENDATIONS

Extensive CVD pathology and increased risk factors can be produced in several animal species via copper deficiency. It is worth noting that copper deficiency does not produce atherosclerosis in any of the animal species tested. Little work has been done on humans, so it is not known how important copper deficiencies are in causing human CVD. Inadequate dietary intakes of copper are common in the U.S. This fact along with the animal work suggests it is prudent to increase dietary copper. This can easily be accomplished by reducing fat, sugar and polished grain consumption and increase whole grains, fresh fruits, shell fish, legumes, green leafy vegetables, lean meats, nuts and seeds. These recommendations are consistent with all other dietary advise on preventing CVD covered in this book. There is no evidence to support megadose copper supplements. Indeed long term supplementation above 5 mg/day has not been tried on humans. If one decides to supplement instead of eating better, then 2 mg of copper per day is a safe and reasonable maximum.

ZINC

Klevay's zinc/copper theory of the cause of CVD states high intakes of zinc and low amounts of copper promote CVD. This theory has tended to stiffle any interest in zinc as a protective factor. Klevay has argued Western diets are too high in zinc but this is not born out by any of the dietary surveys in the United States. A recent investigation concluded 68% of the subjects consumed less than 2/3rds of the RDA for zinc per day. In 1973 Sandstead collected impressive evidence of poor zinc nutrition in large sections of the U. S. population. Even Klevay's survey of copper and zinc intakes showed most diets contained 2/3rds of the RDA or less for zinc. Hence the possibility of high zinc consumption being a factor in CVD incidence in the U. S. is remote. There is no support for the zinc part of the zinc/copper hypothesis.

Serum cholesterol levels in rats were reported by Klevay to be elevated by high zinc/copper ratios. Several animal

studies by others since then have not supported zinc's role
in serum cholesterol elevation. Massive daily doses of zinc
(440 mg zinc sulfate=160 mg zinc) significantly lowered (25%)
high density lipoprotein levels in healthy adult men, but had
no effect on total serum cholesterol. A more recent study on
32 healthy females using 15mg, 50mg and 100mg zinc supplements did not effect plasma HDL levels. Another recent
report showed 29 mg of zinc daily for 8 weeks did not alter
HDL or serum cholesterol in 44 males. These investigations
make it doubtful that moderate zinc supplements have harmful
effects on serum total cholesterol or serum HDL in humans.

Another finding which discouraged interest in zinc's role
in CVD was animals did not exhibit atherosclerosis on zinc
deficient diets. We could summarize the work on animals by
saying there is little evidence supporting a role for zinc
causing or preventing CVD. Nevertheless, clinical trials
using zinc supplements on persons with peripheral vascular
disease did produce a beneficial outcome.

Interest in zinc and atherosclerosis was generated by
Pories' discovery of accelerated wound healing in animals and
humans using zinc supplements. Since atherosclerosis is
probably a "response to injury", this disease can be viewed
as improper wound healing and zinc should promote proper
wound healing. In another finding, Pories showed arteries
have a very high turnover rate of zinc compared to other
tissues. When arteries are injured, the already high zinc
turnover rate is tripled. Also, several investigators
reported substantially lower serum and hair zinc in
atherosclerosis patients in comparison to normals, but it
should be pointed out, serum and hair values are no longer
considered reliable indicators of zinc status. With these
early findings, it is easy to see why clinical trials were
initiated using zinc on advanced perpheral vascular disease
patients.

Pories et .al. in 1967 reported significant improvement in
12 out of 13 patients with inoperable vascular disease given
150 mg zinc per day. Henzel et. al. in 1968 enthusiastically
announced remarkable improvement in 6 out of 10 advanced
peripheral vascular disease patients. Two subjects with
Reynaud's syndrome were greatly benefited as were 4 patients
with intermittent claudication. Increased excercise tolerance and blood flow to the extremities were the common

results. In another trial published by Henzel in 1970, 18 out of 24 subjects with symptomatic atherosclerosis had measureable improvement after taking 150 mg zinc for one year or more. The most common finding was marked reduction of intermittent claudication.

Recently an interesting series of experiments have shown zinc deficiency mimics essential fatty acid deficiency symptoms in rats, including retarded growth, hair loss, skin keratosis and impaired immune response as indicated by atrophy of the thymus. Surprisingly, these symptoms of zinc deficiency in the rat can be eliminated for the most part by supplying dihomo-gamma-linolenic acid but not by linoleic acid.

Linoleic acid is the most commonly available essential fatty acid in vegetable oils. Linoleic acid must first be converted into dihomo-gamma-linolenic acid, a step which requires zinc, in order to have essential fatty acid function. This is the main reason linoleic acid cannot be used to relieve essential fatty acid deficiency if zinc deficits are also present. This also means linoleic acid cannot be used to make prostaglandins when zinc deficiencies are present. Dihomo-gamma-linolenic acid, found in evening primrose oil, does not require zinc in order to make prostaglandins.

There are numerous experiments showing remarkable beneficial effects of certain prostaglandins on the cardiovascular system (see section on prostaglandins), such as reduced platelet aggregation, reduced blood pressure, increased blood flow to the extremities and ischemic ulcer healing when given to patients with advanced peripheral vascular disease. The beneficial effect of supplements on peripheral vascular disease could in large part be due to the requirement for zinc in the conversion of linoleic acid to dihomo-gamma-linolenic acid, thereby permitting the production of "good" prostaglandins.

SUMMARY and RECOMMENDATIONS: ZINC

The theory that excess zinc is a common cause of CVD is not very convincing since most people in the U.S. do not ingest the RDA of zinc. Animals do not demonstrate cardiovascular pathology with either excessive zinc or zinc deficits. There have been conflicting reports on zinc's effect on serum cholesterol, but the most recent human work claim no adverse effects with moderate supplements.

Humans with peripheral vascular disease are benefited by zinc supplements. The benefits are probably due to zinc's important role in wound healing and prostaglandin production. There is no evidence zinc is involved in preventing or causing CVD, but the clinical trials show zinc supplements may help to reverse peripheral vascular disease.

The RDA for zinc is 15 mg. The amounts in most diets range from 6 to 12 mg, indicating many people get inadequate amounts. The reasons for this are the same as for copper and magnesium, that is, diets rich in fat, sugar and polished grains don't have much room left for zinc containing foods. High protein foods, such as meats, seafoods, legumes, whole grains, nuts and seeds, are the best sources of zinc. Four ounce servings of these foods provide from 4 to 6 mg of zinc. The zinc in animal protein is more absorbable than from vegetable protein. Fruits and vegetables are not good sources of zinc.

Zinc supplements for peripheral vascular disease patients would seem to have a favorable risk-reward ratio. The clinical trials used 150 mg. It seems prudent to use considerably less than that if the supplementation goes on for many months due to the fact that zinc inhibits selenium and copper absorption. Selenium and copper deficiencies in animals can be produced by long term excessive zinc supplementation. Routine supplements in healthy persons should not be more than 15 mg daily.

REFERENCES

COPPER

Danks, D. Copper Deficiency in Humans. Ann Rev Nutr 8:235-57,1988

Klevay, L. Copper and ischemic heart disease. Biol Trace Element Res 5:245,1983.

Klevay, L. Dietary Copper: A Powerful Determinant of Cholesterolemia. Med Hypoth 24:111-9,1987

Masironi, R. Trace elements and cardiovascular diseases. WHO Bull 40:305,1969.

Masironi, R. and Shaper, A. Epidemiological studies of health effects of water.   Ann Rev Nutr 1:375-400,1981.

Reiser, S. et. al. Effect of Copper Intake on Blood Cholesterol and lipoprotein. Nutr Rep Int 36:641-9,1987.

ZINC

Black, M. et. al. Zinc supplements and serum lipids in young males.   Am J Clin Nutr 47:970-5,1988.

Crouse, S. et. al. Zinc ingestion and Lipoprotein V in sedentary and endurance-trained men. JAMA 252:785-7,1984.

Freeland-Graves, J. et.al. Effect of zinc supplementation on plasma HDL cholesterol. Am J Clin Nutr 35:988-92,1982

Hambridge, K. M. et. al. Zinc in Trace Elements in Human and Animal Nutrition, Vol 2, 5th ed., Mertz, W. ed. 1987.

Henzel, J. et.al. Efficacy of zinc medication a therapeutic modality in atherosclerosis. Trace Substances in Environmental Health IV D.D. Hemphill ed. 1970

Holden, J. et. al. Zinc and copper in self selected diets. J Am Diet Assn 75:23-8,1979.

Hooper, P. et.al. Zinc lowers HDL cholesterol levels. JAMA 244:1960-1,1980.

Huang, Y. et.al. Most biological effects of zinc deficiency corrected by gamma-linolenic acid. Athero 41:193-207,1982.

Pories, W. et.al. Trace elements and wound healing. Trace Substances in Environmental Health. D.Hemphill ed. 1967.

Sandstead, H. Zinc nutrition in the U. S. Am J Clin Nutr 26:1251-60,1973.

5. CHROMIUM and SELENIUM

ANIMAL EXPERIMENTS: CHROMIUM

A great deal of confusion and uncertainty exists today concerning chromium and human health. The important reviews by Mertz (1969) and Schroeder et. al.(1970) indicate there was little uncertainty in 1970 for either the human or animal work. Mertz summarized the situation with rats and monkeys as follows: 1. Chromium deficiency produces impaired glucose tolerance, elevated serum cholesterol, increased fasting glucose, sugar in the urine, vascular fibrous plaque, decreased growth and decreased longevity. 2. Chromium supplements prevent or reverse these pathological changes, many of which are identical to human adult onset diabetes. Today the animal work could be summarized almost identically.

CHROMIUM CONCENTRATIONS

The uncertainty has primarily arisen in human work due to the wide range of chromium concentrations reported for human tissues, serum and urine and the occasional conflicting results of chromium supplemental trials. In the late 1960's

it appeared as though persons with impaired glucose tolerance
or atherosclerosis had deficient chromium status when
compared to normals. Also, average tissue concentrations in
the United States were reported to be considerably lower than
for persons from countries where diabetes and atherosclerosis
were less prevalent. Many of the tissue values were based on
Schroeder's work. He and others could make a very convincing
case for chromium deficiency as an important risk factor in
human atherosclerosis and diabetes based on 1. the animal
work, 2. the low chromium intakes in the United States,
3. the low chromium tissue concentrations in atherosclerosis, diabetes and the United States population, 4. the
significant improvement occuring in glucose tolerance and
serum lipids, including cholesterol, in human supplemental
chromium trials.

Guthrie's 1982 review has nicely compiled the massive
amount of variable concentration data. The average chromium
concentration in the liver of normal subjects, as reported in
22 different studies, ranged from 9 nanograms(ng) chromium
per gram of wet tissue to 603 ng/gram wet tissue. In 54
published analyses of chromium in serum or plasma, the
reported values ranged evenly from .08 ng/ml to 53 ng/ml (I
have excluded Schroeder's 170ng and 520 ng values). The
recent values for serum are 2 ng or less and the older values
are 10 ng or more. Average urinary chromium excretion for
normal adults in 35 different reports bounces from .3 ng/day
to 42 ng/day. Average hair chromium in 19 different studies
spanned 90 ng/gram to 2450 ng/gram. In 29 published reports
of average dietary intake, the values ranged from 29 micro-
grams/day to 2620 micrograms/day.

This is an unheard of range of figures coming from pres-
tigious and reputable laboratories around the world. Why is
there such a variability in concentrations? One major
reason is contamination from environmental sources of
chromium, especially stainless steel. If, for example, a
wet sample is homogenized with a stainless steel blade, the
chromium concentration increases 21%, but a dry sample
homogenized for one minute increases by 150% and after 3
minutes, a 600% increase! Collecting and storing blood and
tissue samples in stainless steel produces an unknown error.

Another source of error in the earlier (pre 1978) work
was relatively insensitive analytical instruments. When you

consider the reported values are in the nanogram range (one nanogram is one billionth of a gram or one millionth of a milligram), it becomes evident why the instruments need to be extremely sensitive. The earlier instruments gave falsely high and possibly meaningless values.

The chromium concentration in food can vary capriciously even if sensitive instruments are used and sample contamination is avoided, because foods are often contaminated during processing, aging or storage. There is consistent evidence wheat loses a large percentage of its chromium when the germ and bran are removed, but stainless steel grinding equipment can add appreciable amounts when converting it into flour. For example, coarsely ground wheat has a reported value of 13 ng/gram and finely ground wheat, 73 ng/gram. Beer and wine have remarkably high values, 350 ng/gram and 450 ng/gram respectively. These numbers probably reflect contamination from stainless steel containers rather than naturally occuring concentrations.

The contamination of the food supply shed great doubt on any dietary chromium investigation, regardless how perfect the analysis is. What, for example, does the added chromium from stainless steel do for the organism eating the food? It probably doesn't have biological utility. Toepfer et. al. in 1973 found no correlation between a food's chromium content and its biological chromium activity. Beer, which has one of highest concentrations of chromium, has one of the lowest chromium biological activities. A person drinking a quart of beer would have a diet very high in chromium but very low in chromium usability. I think you can appreciate the confusion and uncertainty there is with chromium nutrition and status in humans. It is a confusing situation which deserves urgent scientific attention.

There are many papers reporting lower hair, serum and urinary chromium in diabetics compared to normals, including depressed chromium concentrations after a glucose challenge. Coronary artery disease patients and multiparous women have lower status in published studies also. Since we are well aware of the analysis problems, we should suspend judgement until future reports either confirm or deny the differences.

CLINICAL TRIALS

Fortunately, the most important topic, which is supplemental chromium's effect on CVD risk factors, does not depend on chromium blood, hair, tissue or urine analysis. Two types of chromium supplements have been used on humans. One type is inorganic chromium in the form of chromium chloride. The usual dose given is 150 micrograms, although some experiments have used as much as 1000 micrograms per day. The other supplemental form is the glucose tolerance factor (GTF), a biologically active complex of chromium, amino acids and nicotinic acid. GTF is not a specific compound, but a series of related complexes having biological activity. The dosage of GTF given ranges from 4 to 50 micrograms per day. GTF is absorbed 50 times better and has much higher biological activity than inorganic chromium. Since brewers yeast is the richest natural source of GTF, it is often used in clinical trials and then compared with torula yeast, which contains no chromium or GTF.

A number of studies show significant lowering of serum cholesterol when inorganic chromium or brewers yeast are administered to diabetic or normal subjects. Schroeder in 1968 claimed a 10% lowering in 10 subjects using inorganic chromium. Doisy in 1976 had a 20% fall in 28 subjects using brewers yeast. Nath in 1979 reported a 12% lowering in 12 patients. Offenbacher in 1980 had a 11% decrease in 12 patients with brewers yeast. Elwood in 1982 published a 12% decline using brewers yeast on 27 subjects. Ristes in 1979 and Elwood in 1982 reported significant increases in the beneficial HDL. We can see there is good evidence demonstrating 200 micrograms of inorganic chromium or 10 to twenty grams of brewers yeast significantly lowers serum cholesterol in normals, hyperlipidemics and mildly diabetic patients. HDL levels are probably helped also.

A variety of studies since the 1960's have investigated the effect of chromium or brewers yeast on glucose tolerance. Glinsmann and Mertz's 1966 paper illustrates the trend of the results,in that three of the subjects showed good improvement and three had no improvement. Levine et.al. in 1968 reported four out of ten subjects improved. Doisy et. al. in 1976, using brewers yeast extract claimed six out of twelve benefited. Lui and Morris in 1978 reported seven out of twelve hyperglycemics had marked improvement after taking 5 grams of a brewers yeast extract containing chromium for three months. Nath in 1979 gave 500 micrograms sodium chromate to twelve adult onset diabetics with significant improvement after 9 weeks. Offenbacher and Pi-Sunyer showed improvement in 12 subjects taking brewers yeast. Seventeen out of eighteen mild hyperglycemics had improvement after taking 200 micrograms of chromium for 12 weeks in Polanskys 1981 report. Anderson et. al. claimed 200 micrograms of chromium improved the average glucose tolerance of 35 mild hyperglycemics. Sherman in 1968, in one of the very few negative reports, showed no improvement for 14 diabetics given 150 micrograms of chromium for 16 weeks. In summary, there is mounting evidence demonstrating chromium or brewers yeast improves the glucose tolerance for a large percentage of mild non-insulin dependent diabetics.

An elevated serum insulin level is an important predictor of cardiovascular risk, possibly a more powerful risk factor than serum cholesterol. Tissue culture experiments have shown insulin promotes damage to the endothelium, which provides a sound physiological basis for insulin as a risk factor. Animal and tissue work suggests adequate chromium-GTF should lower serum insulin, since GTF-chromium works with insulin to potentiate its action. A number of reports have shown chromium or brewers yeast supplements lower insulin in normals and diabetics, but the effect is not consistent with several researchers claiming no effects on insulin levels. Lowering serum insulin is an extremely important effect and more research is needed to see if the insulin reductions using chromium are real or chance happenings.

An important trial on diabetics by Rabinowitz et. al. showing no significant improvement with inorganic chromium or brewers yeast was published in 1983. It was a well controlled 4 month trial with no benefits for serum cholesterol, triglycerides, insulin or glucose tolerance. A major difference in this trial, when compared to the numerous sucessful ones cited above, is the severity of the diabetes. For example, the fasting glucose levels in the sucessful trials ranged around 100 mg/100 ml or slightly above and the patients were not insulin dependent, but in Rabinowitz's experiment, the subjects fasting glucose averaged around 200 mg/100 ml and they were insulin dependent. Even though

Rabinowitz's group was considerably sicker, they received considerably less brewers yeast than in most trials (6.8grams vs 11 to 50 grams in other trials). One positive result overlooked by Rabinowitz was the consistent 5 to 17% decline in fasting glucose in those subjects taking chromium or brewers yeast. This study suggests frank diabetics are not helped very much with four months of minimal chromium or brewers yeast supplements. On the other hand many previous experiments conclude mild diabetics are benefited by chromium or brewers yeast supplements.

SUMMARY and RECOMMENDATIONS: CHROMIUM

Chromium deficiencies produce adult onset diabetes in animals. All the symptoms occur, such as poor glucose tolerance, elevated serum lipids, and some atherosclerosis. Chromium is an essential part of a molecular complex named glucose tolerance factor (GTF). GTF appears to be necessary for proper insulin function and glucose metabolism.

Food and tissue chromium concentrations published before 1978 are probably incorrect. This makes all the early discussions on human chromium status and deficient diets of uncertain value. Clinical trials using chromium supplements show 40 to 60% of the non-insulin dependent diabetics respond with lower serum lipids and improved glucose tolerance.

Our dietary recommendations are the same for chromium as for the other nutrients. Fat, sugar and polished grains have less chromium and whole grains, legumes, fruits and vegetables have more chromium. Reliable food value tables are not available at this time. The tentative RDA of 40 to 200 ug is probably incorrect due to unreliable analyses. Some clinical trials report theraputic benefits with only 25 ug or several tablespoons of brewers yeast, which suggests the RDA is too high.

The risk-reward ratio for supplementing with chromium is not as favorable as for magnesium because of the great uncertainty concerning optimum intake. This is critical for trace elements, because their range of safety is much smaller. Since some clinical trials sucessfully used 25 to 50 ug, this seems a reasonable upper limit for chronic supplementation. Better yet, 2 to 3 tablespoons of Brewers yeast produces clinical benefit. Brewers yeast makes sense because it is a nutrient rich food, especially for chromium and vitamin B-6.

SELENIUM

Selenium, along with vitamin E are antioxidants. Together they help prevent the auto-oxidation (peroxidation) of lipids. Polyunsaturated fats are unusually susceptable to peroxidation by oxygen and hydrogen peroxide. Since polyunsaturated fats are components of all cell membranes and cell organelle membranes such as mitochondria and ribosomes, it is easy to see why cells and cell organelles are damaged by peroxidation.

Free radicals and malonaldehyde are breakdown products of lipid peroxides, both of which react with DNA, protein and polyunsaturated fats, often forming large, complicated polymers. One such polymer is lipofuscin, a yellowish-brown randomly assembled, complex molecule composed of polyunsaturated fat and protein. Lipofuscin, sometimes called age pigment, accumulates with age in cells, especially around the nuclei of myocardial fibers.

Lipid auto-oxidation has been implicated in atherosclerosis and myocardial fibrosis for some time. There is a close parallel between the amount of aortic atheroma present and lipid auto-oxidation products in arterial plaque. Human atherosclerotic plaques have been found to contain oxidation products of linoleic acid, the most common polyunsaturated fat. In fact, aortic lesions and myocardial fibrosis can be produced in rabbits by subcutaneous administration of linoleate hydroperoxide, the auto-oxidation product of linoleic acid. Selenium treatment has been shown to inhibit and prevent myocardial lipid oxidation and subsequent myocardial damage. Age pigment can be prevented or inhibited by a variety of antioxidants including selenium and vitamin E.

Adriamycin (doxorubicin), an effective cancer chemotheraputic drug, has an unfortunate side effect of heart muscle degeneration including fibrosis. Adriamycin is a powerful oxidant, causing lipid peroxidation and malonaldehyde formation. The heart muscle degeneration is caused by the lipid peroxidation and malonaldehyde. In animal work, antioxidants such as vitamin E and selenium, sharply reduce the heart muscle degeneration induced by adriamycin. There is also less malonaldehyde and lipid peroxidation when selenium or other antioxidants are given with adriamycin. The work with adriamycin adds substantial support to the notion that lipid peroxidation is an important factor in heart muscle degeneration. Antioxidants sharply reduce this cause of heart muscle degeneration.

Mammals on a selenium deficient diet, without added oxidation stresses, develop heart and striated muscle degeneration. The cardiac lesions are usually subendocardial, grayish-white plaques. In addition, characteristic electrocardiogram abnormalities occur, such as an elevated S-T segment, similar to that seen in human myocardial infarction. Animals with selenium deficiency induced heart muscle degeneration have a high incidence of sudden heart death. Also, a capillary degeneration in chickens, called exudative diathesis is produced by selenium deficient regimens.

HUMAN STUDIES: SELENIUM

Epidemiology supports the idea that selenium deficiency is a risk factor in cardiovascular disease. Areas in the United States with high selenium content of forage crops have significantly lower CVD death rate than in low selenium areas. States with the highest selenium concentrations in drinking water have the lowest hypertensive death rate. A study in 17 matched cities in high and low selenium areas, showed significantly lower CVD death rates in high selenium cities. In another study, the mean blood bank selenium levels were inversely correlated with CVD death rate. A study in high and low selenium areas in Finland revealed selenium as a statistically significant protective factor also. Further, the calculated dietary selenium intake in 25 countries was inversely correlated with CVD death rate in those countries.

An important prospective case-control study in Finland recently reported lower serum selenium levels in persons experiencing myocardial infarct or dying from cardiovascular disease than matched controls. The relative risk of coronary death was 6.9 times greater in persons with serum selenium below 34 ug/ml compared to persons above 45 ug/ml. A similar relative risk was found for all cardiovascular deaths. It should be noted serum levels in the United States are usually above 100 ug/ml.

A controlled investigation in Germany reported lower platelet glutathione peroxidase, an important selenium dependent enzyme, in patients with acute myocardial infarct. There is well grounded speculation that adequate selenium should favor reduced platelet aggregation for two reasons: 1. Anti-oxidants like selenium reduce lipid peroxide concentrations and lipid peroxides inhibit prostacyclin production, the powerful anti-aggregating prostaglandin. 2. There is some evidence that anti-oxidants increase the production of good prostaglandins.

Recently, cultured endothelial cells supplied with selenium had up to three times higher prostacyclin production than unsupplemented cells. In the same study, selenium supplements in five volunteers doubled the average bleeding time (indicating greater platelet stability) after six weeks. This trial confirms the speculation on selenium's beneficial effect on platelets.

There have been two small trials using vitamin E and selenium on angina patients reporting reduced angina and increased exercise tolerance. There has been one large controlled trial using selenium in China to prevent a heart muscle degeneration called Keshan disease. This is probably the largest controlled trial ever performed using a vitamin or mineral as the variable. Keshan disease is a cardiomyopathy featuring fibrosis and multiple focal myocardial necrosis. It is most commonly found in children under 15 years of age and the usual cause of death is congestive heart failure. Keshan disease occurs in low selenium soil areas and victims have very low serum selenium values. Selenium supplements dramatically reduced both the incidence and death rate due to Keshan disease. There were 36,603 selenium supplemented children and 9642 controls. During the four year investigation, 21 cases and 3 deaths occured in the treated group, but there were 107 cases and 53 deaths in the control group, which was a 20 fold lower case rate and a 70 fold lower death rate in the treated group.

Unlike most minerals, soil selenium levels are directly reflected in food crop concentrations. If one is eating all his food grown or raised in a low selenium area, the dietary intake of selenium will be low, regardless of what is eaten. In the United States, transport of food grown in high selenium areas to low selenium areas helps to moderate the deficiencies in low selenium areas. There is little food transportation in China, hence areas with low soil selenium eat selenium poor food exclusively. Also, wheat which is a selenium accumulator and usually has higher selenium concentrations than other foods, is more commonly eaten in the U. S. than China. Both of these factors account for the rarity of pure Keshan disease in the U. S. even in low selenium soil areas. Nevertheless, low selenium areas in the U. S. do have higher CVD death rates than high selenium areas.

SUMMARY and RECOMMENDATIONS: SELENIUM

Animal work shows heart muscle degeneration, abnormal electrocardiograms, and increased auto-oxidation damage of polyunsaturated fats occurs on selenium deficient regimens. In humans, a syndrome of heart muscle degeneration is found in low selenium areas and is prevented with selenium supplements. National and international epidemiology plus case control studies supports a selenium rich diet as a protective factor and a poor selenium diet as a risk factor. Certainly the case for selenium deficiency being a major cause of CVD in the U.S. has not been proved, but the evidence is strong enough to encourage a prudent man to consume adequate amounts of high selenium foods.

The average intake of selenium in the U.S. is around 100 ug (micrograms), compared to 300 ug in Japan. We have less selenium in our diets than countries with low rates of CVD. The reason for our selenium poor diets is fat, sugar and polished grains contain very little selenium. Seafoods and whole grains, especially whole wheat, are the best sources of selenium. Four ounces of seafood has up to 100 ug and four ounces of whole wheat flour has up to 80 ug of selenium. In order to have a selenium rich diet, our food recommendations are similar to those found in other sections of this book, that is, replace fat, sugar and polished grains with nutrient rich foods such as whole wheat and seafoods. Unfortunately, fruits and vegetables are poor sources of selenium.

The tentative RDA by the National Research Council for selenium is 50-200 ug. International epidemiology suggests up to 300 ug is a safe range. By eliminating fat, sugar and polished grains and including more seafoods and whole grains, daily amounts in the range of 200-300 ug can be expected. Supplements are available for people with poor diets. In no case should you supplement with more than 200 ug per day because little is known about excessive consumption of selenium. As with all trace elements, megadoses are toxic.

REFERENCES

CHROMIUM

Anderson,R. Chromium in Trace Elements in Human & Animal Nutrition, 5th ed, Vol 1, p225-44, Mertz, ed.1987

Anderson, R & Kozlovsky, A. Chromium intake, absorption & excretion. Am J Clin Nutr 41:1177-83,1985

Anderson, R. et. al. Effect of chromium supplements on subjects with marginally elevated or depressed blood glucose following a glucose load. Am J Clin Nutr 35:840,1982

Elwood, J. et. al. Effect of high chromium brewers yeast on human serum lipids. J Am Col Nutr 1:263-74,1982

Guthrie, B. "Nutritional role of chromium" in Biological and environmental aspects of chromium. Langard(ed) Elsevier Biomedical Press 1982 pp.117-148.

Mertz, W. Chromium occurence and function in biological systems. Physiological Reviews 49,163-239,1969.

Offenbacher, E. & Pi-Sunyer, Chromium in Human Nutrition, Ann Rev Nutr 8:543-63,1988

Potter, J. et. al. Glucose Metab. in Glucose Intolerant older people during Chromium Supple. Metab 34:199-204,1985.

Rabinowitz, M. et. al. Effects of chromium and yeast supplements on carbohydrate and lipid metabolism in diabetic men. Diabetes Care 6:319-27,1983

Schroeder, H. et. al. Chromium deficiency as a factor in atherosclerosis. J Chronic Dis 23:123-42,1970.

Shapcott & Hubert, eds. Chromium in Nutrition and Metabolism. Elsevier New York. 1979. Contains many original papers.

SELENIUM

Chen, X. et.al. Studies on the relations of selenium and Keshan disease. Biol Trace Elem Res 2:91-107,1980.

Frost,D. The two faces of selenium–can selenophobia be cured? CRC Crit Rev Tox 1:467-514,1972.

Levander, O. A Global View of Human Selenium Nutrition. Ann Rev Nutr 7:227-50,1987.

Salonen, J. et.al. Association between cardiovascular death and myocardial infarction and serum selenium in a matched-pair longitudinal study. Lancet 2:175-9,1982.

Schiavon, R. et.al. Selenium enhances prostacyclin production by cultured endothelial cells. Thrombosis Research 34: 389-396,1984.

Shamberger, R. Biochemistry of Selenium. Plenum Press. New York. 1983.

Shamberger, R. et.al. Selenium and heart disease II. in Trace Substances in Environmental Health, vol 12, 1978, pp 48-52.

Wang,Y. et.al. Selenium and myocardial infarction:glutathione peroxidase in platelets. Klin Wochenschr 59:817-8,1981.

6. VITAMIN B6 and VITAMIN C

VITAMIN B6

Vitamin B6 is a water soluble vitamin involved in a large number of enzymatic processes. There are three naturally occuring varieties. Pyridoxine, a heat stable form, is found in plants. Pyridoxal and pyridoxamine are forms found in animals and are sensitive to heat and ultraviolet light. These three forms are converted in the body into pyridoxal phosphate, a co-enzyme for many biochemical reactions. Vitamin B6 is required in a great many essential reactions in protein and amino acid metabolism. In addition, several important steps in carbohydrate metabolism require B6. For example, the conversion of glycogen into glucose phosphate by liver and muscle requires B6. Also, without B6, linoleic acid can not function as an essential fatty acid or as a precursor for prostaglandins.

ATHEROSCLEROSIS

The first reports of vitamin B6 deficiency producing cardiovascular abnormalities in animals appeared in the early 1940's. Cardiac hypertrophy occured in almost all the rats, dogs and hogs tested, along with a high percentage of myocarditis and mural thrombosis. This work was confirmed in the

1960's and most recently in 1979. There are, in addition, profound electrocardiographic abnormalities in B6 deficient animals.

In 1949, Rinehart and Greenberg reported monkeys on B6 poor diets, which were also low in fat and cholesterol, developed atherosclerosis. The monkeys arteries exhibited proliferation of smooth muscle cells, production of excessive amounts of connective tissue, fibrous material and matrix which resulted in greatly thickened intima. Rinehart and Greenberg, who were both pathologists at the University of California San Francisco Medical Center, claimed the lesions looked remarkably similar to human fibrous plaque except for the lack of lipid infiltration. The location of the plaque in the arteries was similar to the human condition. When cholesterol was added to the diet, serum cholesterol was markedly elevated, especially when compared to controls on adequate vitamin B6. The added cholesterol did not appear to increase lipid infiltration of the lesions, but calcification of the arteries was occasionally noted. Rinehart and Greenberg repeated and confirmed their results several times as did Muskett and Emerson in 1956 and later Kuzuya. In 1978 it was reported the effects of moderate copper deficiency is made worse by B6 deficits, with resulting degeneration of arterial elastin.

One group of researchers, Mann and Stare, did not report atherosclerosis in B6 deficient monkeys, but they had very few animals in their experiments, for example, there was only one monkey in their first experiment. Most important, the monkeys were so profoundly B6 deficient that they did not live long enough to develop atherosclerosis.

HOMOCYSTINE

Homocystine research supports the studies on B6 deficiencies and atherosclerosis. Animal and human work have shown homocystine accumulates on low B6 diets. When given intravenously to rabbits, monkeys or baboons, homocystine produces extensive atherosclerosis and thrombosis. Many careful investigations have demonstrated homocystine severely damages the endothelium. In baboons given intravenous homocystine, 10% of the aortic surface was deendothelialized even though there was a 25 fold increase in endothelial cell regeneration. All of the animals given homocystine developed atherosclerotic or pre-atherosclerotic lesions.

A well known way to generate atherosclerosis in animals is to damage the endothelium by chemical or physical means. After the endothelium is damaged, platelets are activated, releasing chemicals which cause smooth muscle proliferation and thickened intima leading to fibrous plaque. When platelet stabilizers are given to animals with damaged endothelium, fibrous plaque does not develop, indicating the profound role platelets play in atherosclerosis. When homocystine and platelet stabilizers are given together, damaged endothelium occurs, but no vascular lesions are produced. Experimenters have concluded that homocystine promotes atherosclerosis by damaging endothelium.

Persons with a rare inherited syndrome called homocystinuria, characterized by high blood levels of homocystine, usually die at a young age with advanced atherosclerosis and thromboembolism. It is likely the high blood levels of homocystine causes the atherosclerosis and thromboembolism. The reason for the high blood level of homocystine was uncovered a number of years ago. It goes something like this: Methionine is a sulfur containing amino acid which goes through a number of transformations when it is metabolized. One metabolite produced is called homocysteine which is subsequently converted into cystathionine by a vitamin B6 dependent enzyme named cystathionine synthase. If this enzyme is missing or defective, homocysteine is blocked in its normal transformation to cystathionine and is converted into homocystine instead. There are two forms of this disease. One type completely lacks the enzyme and the other variant has a defective enzyme. Patients with a defective enzyme are helped with high doses of vitamin B6.

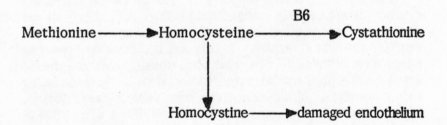

Another way to impair cystathionine synthase activity and produce homocystine is to reduce the availability of vitamin B6. In experiments done on humans by Park and Linkswiler, it was shown high protein diets (150 grams) coupled with low B6 intake (.16 mg) resulted in homocystine excretion. It took 2.2 mg of B6 to prevent the homocystine excretion in most persons. All of the B6 deficient subjects excreted homocystine when given an oral dose of methionine.

In a study done in 1976 by Wilkins and Wilkins, it was reported coronary artery disease patients respond to a load of methionine with higher cysteine-homocysteine blood levels than normals. The above work suggests an important link between B6 deficiencies and atherosclerosis is homocystine production. Excessive animal protein, which contains much more methionine than vegetable protein, coupled with low vitamin B6 diets makes this occurance more likely.

In 1985 Boers et. al. found 30% of their premature peripheral vascular and cerebral occlusive arterial disease patients were heterozygotes for homocystinuria. These authors considered their elevated homocysteine levels to be an important factor in the development of their premature vascular disease. Israelsson et. al. in 1988 reported a high incidence (24%) of myocardial infarct patients with high plasma homocysteine as their only risk factor.

Another interesting line of investigation has revealed Downs Syndrome patients on autopsy are free of atherosclerosis. They also have significantly lower plasma homocysteine levels because of the enzyme abnormalities found in these patients. A number of authors have suggested the low homocysteine level is the likely reason for the reduced incidence of atherosclerosis.

PLATELET AGGREGATION

Recently it was discovered vitamin B6 is an important anti-thrombogenic agent. Thrombus formation is a complex multistep process. Platelets exposed to collagen and subendothelial tissue initiates the first phase of platelet aggregation, where ADP (adinosine diphosphate) and the prostaglandin thromboxane A-2 are released, both of which cause platelets to change shape and adhere to each other.

The second important phase is the release of thrombin for the stabilization and growth of the thrombus. Adrenalin, a hormone associated with stress and increased clotting tendency, potentiates all the steps in thrombus formation. When vitamin B6 (pyridoxal-5-phosphate) is added to a platelet rich media containing ADP, thrombin or adrenalin, the second phase of platelet aggregation was completely inhibited. When the platelets with added B6 were exposed to collagen, ADP and thrombin, the first phase of platelet aggregation was completely abolished. Vitamin B6 inhibits both the first and second phase of platelet aggregation.

Two specific actions of vitamin B6 (pyridoxal-5-phosphate or PALP) on platelets have been uncovered to account for B6's powerful inhibition of platelet aggregation. First, PALP binds with specific platelet surface proteins, thereby interfering with aggregation. Second, PALP increases the cyclic AMP levels in platelets. High cyclic AMP levels have been found to inhibit platelets clotting function.

Intravenous administration of PALP in healthy human volunteers inhibited platelet aggregation, whole blood clotting and thrombin clotting time. In addition to combining with platelet surface proteins, PALP binds with thrombin and fibrinogen. PALP bound thrombin resulted in clotting periods three times longer than controls. A similar decrease in clotting activity occurs with PALP bound fibrinogen. The work published so far lends powerful support for the inhibition of platelet aggregation and clotting by vitamin B6, although a recent paper by Schoene reported vitamin B-6 supplements only produced very mild platelet effects in volunteers.

The potential importance of platelet stabilization in retarding atherosclerosis indeed could be very great. Animals, such as monkeys, dogs and rabbits, whose endothelium is repeatedly damaged develop classic fibrous plaque, including smooth muscle proliferation, excess connective tissue and lipid infiltration. In these same animals, if they are given platelet stabilizers while the endothelium is damaged, atherosclerosis does not result. In the experiments with homocystine, if platelet stabilizers are given along with the homocystine, no atherosclerotic lesions emerge, even though the homocystine causes extensive endothelial damage.

We now have two powerful ways in which vitamin B6 helps prevent atherosclerosis. First, vitamin B6 stabilizes platelets, inhibits their aggregation and clotting. Second, vitamin B6 is essential to prevent the formation of homocystine. These well established functions along with the early and repeated observations that B6 deficiencies in monkeys and dogs results in atherosclerosis, makes it highly likely that vitamin B6 deficiency is a risk factor for cardiovascular disease in humans.

DIETARY INTAKE and NUTRITIONAL STATUS

It has been almost 40 years since Rinehart and Greenberg published their provocative experiments on monkeys and there are still no prospective studies on B6 intake or status and cardiovascular disease. Willett has indicated a prospective study has been initiated, so in the future we may have more decisive data.

There have been few surveys of B6 status and ischemic heart disease. A Russian abstract in 1966 revealed low B6 status in heart disease patients compared to controls but few details were given. Serfontein reported recent myocardial infarct patients had one half the B6 status compared to healthy controls. Rossouw only found mild differences between heart disease patients and controls, but their patients had been on special lipid lowering diets for 3 years which would invalidate any meaningful comparison with controls. It is interesting to note Rossouw reported 31% of their patients and controls were B6 deficient.

A study of 617 men revealed vitamin B6 status decreases with age in men not taking B6 supplements. Decreased status with age has been a consistent finding in other smaller studies. In the group of men not taking supplements, 25 to 30% were classified as having marginal to inadequate B6 status, whereas the group taking supplements had average plasma B6 levels 65% higher. B6 status did not decrease with age in the supplementing group, indicating declining status is not a natural consequence of age.

A survey of 102 hospitalized geriatric patients reported 80% consumed less than half of the 2.2 mg RDA for vitamin B6. Not one of the patients (none of them were critically ill) ate foods providing the RDA for B6. Even though the intakes were remarkably low, the authors argued for a higher

RDA for the aged. Paul Gyorgy, the discoverer of B6 has also proposed a higher RDA for B6.

Schroeder has estimated the typical hospital diet (2400 calories) provides only 0.46 mg to 1.53 mg of B6 per day, with none of them equaling the RDA. A survey of more than 100 female adolescents reported over one half consumed less than 2/3rds of the RDA and 31% exhibited inadequate B6 status. These findings are typical, with a number of other surveys showing mean intakes of 1.3 to 1.6 mg per day. There is good support for the notion that B6 intake and status is not adequate in a large percentage of our population.

The reason for the widespread B6 deficiency is not hard to find. Fat and sugar are devoid of B6, but they comprise 38% and 14% of our calories, respectively. Polished grains, another 20% of our caloric intake, have lost 60% of their original B6. Canned fruits, vegetables and meats usually show losses of 50% when compared to fresh products. The animal form (pyridoxal) is much more heat sensitive than the vegetable form (pyridoxine), but both have equally high water losses because B6 is water soluble.

The best sources of B6 are whole grains, fruits, fresh meats and vegetables, nuts and seeds. The B6 content of a 1/4 pound serving of each food is:

chicken	.55mg	soy flour	.66
beef	.55	whole wheat flour	.37
banana	.55	white wheat flour	.06
potato	.28	wheat germ	1.25
spinach	.31	sunflower seeds	1.36
broccoli	.20	tomato juice	.20
kidney beans	.30	turnip greens	.28
buckwheat flour	.62	brown rice	.60
brewers yeast	4.00	polished rice	.17
fish	.50	walnuts	.80

SUMMARY AND RECOMMENDATIONS: VITAMIN B6

Animals develop atherosclerosis on low vitamin B6 diets. Two mechanisms have been discovered to account for this pathology. First, homocystine accumulates on B6 deficient diets. Homocystine damages endothelium and produces fibrous plaque in animals. Second, vitamin B6 is a platelet stabilizer. Stable platelets inhibit atherosclerosis, unstable platelets promote atherosclerosis. The evidence is compelling enough to convince a prudent person to consume foods rich in vitamin B6. Translated into diet this means restricted amounts of fat, sugar and polished grains but generous portions of vegetables, fruits, whole grains and legumes. Nuts, seeds, and fresh meats contain good amounts of B6, but they are high in fat so they should be used less generously.

The risk-reward ratio is favorable for persons interested in supplementing. Vitamin B6 is very safe at low doses. Patients have taken 50 mg for years without side effects. Women taking 2000 to 6000 mg of B6 for many years did develop peripheral nerve dysfunction, so at massive doses B6 does have dangerous side effects. We are not concerned with megadoses here because supplements in the range of 3 to 10 mg are sufficient to inhibit homocystine formation and stabilize platelets. At these doses the risks are extremely low, the possible rewards are high. If supplements above 50 mg but below 100 mg are taken long term, the risks of side effects, even though small, do go up. It is imprudent to chronically supplement with more than 100 mg per day because of possible risks of sensory nerve dysfunction.

VITAMIN C

There is great popular interest in vitamin C as a prophylactic for colds, flu and cancer plus as an agent for treating these maladies. There are widely divergent opinions, results, interpretations and conclusions on vitamin C for colds, flu and cancer, but at this time it appears ascorbic acid is not particularly effective against these diseases. More research needs to be done before the conflicting results can be resolved completely. In contrast, there is scant popular discussion of vitamin C for prophylaxis or treatment cardiovascular disease, even though there is consistent evidence supporting ascorbic acid as a protective factor for CVD.

ANIMAL MODELS

Vitamin C, strangely enough, is not a vitamin for the majority of vertebrates, since most animals synthesize ascorbic acid from glucose. A dietary source of vitamin C is not required by organisms making their own. Dogs, rats, and rabbits, for example, do not require dietary ascorbic acid, hence vitamin C deficiency studies on these animals are meaningless. Atherosclerosis and CVD risk factors such as serum cholesterol and triglyceride levels are not affected in these animals by varying vitamin C intake.

Guinea pigs, certain birds, fruit eating bats and all primates, including man, have lost the abiltiy to synthesize vitamin C and depend on a constant dietary source. Death results in these animals (and humans of course) if dietary vitamin C is withheld long enough. The course of scurvy leading to death is rapid in guinea pigs, requiring about 4 weeks on a vitamin C free diet. After 2 weeks without vitamin C, guinea pigs rapidly decrease their food consumption and after 3 weeks eating ceases. There is rapid weight loss, negative nitrogen balance, hemorrhaging and multiple nutrient deficiencies. The terminal stage of scurvy is a complicated metabolic derangement and not merely a simple condition of vitamin C deficiency.

There are many divergent reports on lipid metabolism changes in animals during acute scurvy. Some studies report reduced tissue lipid levels, some claim elevations and others see no change. Serum and tissue levels of cholesterol during scurvy have the same confusing results. In men developing scurvy, serum cholesterol stays the same or declines moderately, but after vitamin C supplementation in these subjects, rises somewhat. Since scurvy is a rare condition in Western societies, there are few compelling reasons to apply these results to the etiology of CVD or to work hard to resolve the discrepancies. The uneven results are probably a reflection of the profound and complicated metabolic derangement in scurvy.

An animal model more accurately reflecting the human condition in western societies is latent chronic vitamin C deficiency or what Ginter, a leader in ascorbic acid research, calls hypovitaminosis C. This condition is produced in guinea pigs by putting them on a vitamin C free diet for 2 weeks to deplete the tissue stores and then maintaining them on 0.5 mg of vitamin C per day. Guinea pigs can be kept on this regimen for over a year with no change in weight, appearance or behavior. Interestingly, hypovitaminosis C produces profound changes in the guinea pig cardiovascular system. Serum cholesterol remains fairly constant for the first month or two, but usually by the third month significant rises have occured which are sustained or gradually increase over time. In a series of controlled trials on over 100 animals, Ginter in 1975 found an average 42% increase in serum cholesterol after 20 weeks on a hypovitaminosis C diet. Later work showed increases in the range of 75 to 100%. The cholesterol concentration in the liver of these animals increased also.

Ginter and others have done carbon-14 studies to determine the mechanism behind the increased serum and liver cholesterol concentrations. Repeated experiments demonstrate no increase in the rate of cholesterol synthesis, but there was a 30% decrease in the conversion rate of cholesterol to cholic acid, one of the components of bile. Since the liver makes considerable cholesterol and relatively little is used for cell membranes and steroid hormone manufacture, there are large amounts left over to be excreted. The main mechanism for cholesterol excretion is to convert it into cholic acid, which is excreted as a component of bile. Vitamin C is needed for the transformation of cholesterol into cholic acid. The decrease in the conversion rate of cholesterol into cholic acid appears to be the main reason for the rise in serum cholesterol during hypovitaminosis C.

Another change occuring during hypovitaminosis C is an increase in harmful LDL and a decrease in beneficial HDL, both of which are important human CVD risk factors. It should be emphasized these experiments used low fat, low cholesterol diets. When moderate fat and cholesterol were added, there were greater increases in serum cholesterol.

Guinea pig triglyceride levels are affected adversely during hypovitaminosis C. After several weeks on low fat, cholesterol free, hypovitaminosis C diets, there are gradual increases in serum triglycerides. If saturated fat and cholesterol are included in the diet, then extremely high triglyceride values result, with fat accumulations in the liver and arteries. Subsequent supplementation with ascorbic acid produced marked decreases in serum fat levels. The reasons for ascorbic acid's effect on triglycerides have not been elucidated yet, but it appears depressed enzyme lipoprotein lipase activity is a likely culprit.

An important recent experiment on cultured arterial smooth muscle cells demonstrated ascorbate increased the number of LDL receptors in these cells, causing a 2 to 3 fold increase in LDL degradation rate. Serum LDL is a significant risk factor, with the number of LDL receptors controlling the LDL serum levels. The greater the number of LDL receptors, the lower the serum LDL. Persons with familial hypercholesterolemia lack LDL receptors, which accounts for their exceedingly high serum LDL values. The finding on vitamin C's ability to increase LDL receptors, if confirmed, is an exciting link in our understanding of vitamin C and abnormal lipid metabolism.

ARTERIAL WALL

Collagen is the most prevalent protein in the body, being an important structural molecule in almost all connective tissue, including blood vessel walls. The synthesis of collagen requires vitamin C and as expected there is a decrease in the collagen content of most tissues during vitamin C restriction. Blood vessels may be an exception to this for two reasons. First, blood vessel vitamin C in guinea pigs takes longer to deplete than other tissues. For example, after 9 months on a hypovitaminosis C diet, aorta ascorbic acid concentration was cut by 50% but other tissues lost over 85%. Second, high serum cholesterol and cholesterol deposition in arteries stimulates collagen synthesis. On marginal vitamin C diets, Ginter was unable to demonstrate arterial collagen loss, but previous work by others did. This important issue needs to be resolved.

The glycosaminoglycans (mucopolysaccharides), the complex components of connective tissue important for cardiovascular health, are influenced by vitamin C status. Chrondroitin-4-sulfate (CSA), a glycosaminoglycan, when given orally or intravenously prevents and regresses experimentally induced and naturally occuring atherosclerosis in a variety of animals. The glycosaminoglycans benefit lipid metabolism, inhibit clot and thrombus formation and are needed for the integrity of the connections of the endothelial cells. Animals fed atherogenic diets or guinea pigs fed vitamin C restricted diets result in significant decreases in arterial glycosaminoglycan content, including CSA. In addition, there are increases in the activities of the enzymes which degrade the glycosaminoglycans, namely, B-glucuronidase, B-hexosaminidase, and hyaluronidase. Vitamin C supplements depress these enzymes and restores the glycosaminoglycan content of arteries in a variety of animals.

In summary, there are three reasons why vitamin C deficiency should impair arterial wall health. First, serum cholesterol and triglyceride levels are increased. Second, arterial collegen synthesis may be restricted. Third, glycosaminoglycan content, including CSA, is decreased. Let's look at what happens to arteries on marginal vitamin C regimens.

Weekly changes in arterial tissue in hypovitaminosis C guinea pigs on cholesterol free diets have been published. During the first week, visible wrinkles appear on the endothelium. Endothelial damage and loss begins after the second week, exposing arterial connective tissue. Platelet aggregation and fibrin deposition are triggered by the exposed connective tissue. After eight weeks, Ginter in 1978 noted, "the lesions consisted of fibrous thickening of the intima, with lipid accumulation and degenerative changes in the media accompanied by mucopolysaccharide, lipid and calcium deposits." Edema of the blood vessel wall along with large intimal musculofibrotic plaques also occured. Guinea pigs given moderate dietary cholesterol along with vitamin C restriction develop advanced atheromas "recalling more or less human atherosclerosis." Vitamin C supplements greatly retarded the dietary cholesterol induced atherosclerosis.

The above animal work makes a credible case for the protective effect of adequate vitamin C. Two more topics can be briefly added here. One is vitamin C is required for the synthesis of carnitine, a molecule necessary for fat metabolism in heart and other muscles. Second, Horobin has pointed out vitamin C is probably needed for production of PGE-1, a beneficial, anti-aggregating prostaglandin made by platelets.

EPIDEMIOLOGY

Ginter noted industrial vitamin C production in the United States since 1958 has a remarkable inverse correlation with ischemic heart disease death rate. There has been a steady increase in vitamin C output, particularly dramatic since 1967 and death rates have been dropping rapidly since 1968.

The major dietary source of vitamin C, of course, is fresh fruits and vegetables. Fruit and vegetable consumption has increased in the United States since 1968, corresponding to our decreasing heart disease death rate. Coronary mortality in a 20 country study has a significant inverse correlation with fruit and vegetable consumption. In another 30 nation report, a significant negative correlation was found between vegetable and grain intake and coronary heart disease mortality. In England there is a significant negative correlation between vitamin C intake and CVD death rate. A similar relationship was found in 9 regions of England, Wales and Scotland.

An inverse relationship between vitamin C status or consumption and serum cholesterol values has been reported in many surveys. Seasonal serum cholesterol fluctuations relate inversely with seasonal changes in vitamin C intake. Other surveys demonstrate serum ascorbate is low when serum cholesterol is high. In healthy blood donors, there were three times as many serum cholesterol elevations with low vitamin C values than with high vitamin C levels. HDL levels have an apparent inverse relationship with leucocyte ascorbate concentration. Also, coronary artery disease patients have substantially lower ascorbate concentrations than patients without coronary artery disease. The epidemiology and surveys reported solidly support adequate vitamin C as a protective factor and vitamin C deficiency as a CVD risk factor. Remember, epidemiology only suggests or supports a relationship, it can never prove a linkage.

CLINICAL TRIALS

One of the first series of controlled trials was done by Sokoloff et. al. in 1967. They reported significant serum cholesterol and triglyceride reductions in 122 patients, compared to 55 placebo controls, when given 2 grams of ascorbic acid for 6 to 24 months. The younger patients with initial serum cholesterol below 250 showed little change. This is in line with many other trials demonstrating vitamin C does not lower serum cholesterol in persons with normal inital values. Sokoloff's other patients with serum cholesterol above 275 had average serum cholesterol lowering of 18 to 25%. There was an even greater fall in average triglyceride of 36 to 50%.

In 1979 Ginter resolved the conflicting results which were beginning to appear in the literature. He reviewed thirteen published trials and found the serum cholesterol response to vitamin C is a function of initial cholesterol values. He found serum cholesterol values below 200 mg% did not respond to vitamin C supplements, but above that value there was usually clear benefit, with the greater the initial value the greater the benefit. Seven controlled clinical trials have demonstrated vitamin C supplements above 500 mg/day produce hypocholesterolemic effects in groups with initial serum cholesterol above 200 mg%. Also, patients with poor initial vitamin C status respond better than patients with good initial status. Serum cholesterol lowering with vitamin C usually takes a minimum of 2 months.

Bordia in 1980 reported 2 grams of vitamin C daily increased the fibrinolytic activity by 50% and decreased platlet adhesiveness in myocardial infarct patients. Serum cholesterol was lowered 12% and HDL increased, but not significantly. Heine and Norden gave 1 gram vitamin C for an average of 16 months to 63 peripheral vascular disease patients with elevated serum cholesterol. Serum cholesterol was lowered an average of 11%, but serum triglyceride was not significantly reduced. They did report a noteworthy rise in HDL from 41 to 56 mg%.

Spittle in 1973 dramatically reduced deep vein thrombosis in surgical patients in a controlled trial using one gram of vitamin C per day. Dr. Spittle now routinely administers one gram of vitamin C daily on the surgical and burn wards and claims to have eliminated deep vein thrombosis as a surgical complication. Complimenting the clinical trials is the reported requirement for vitamin C in the synthesis of PGE-1, a beneficial antiaggregating prostaglandin.

It has been known since 1972 that after a myocardial infarct, leucocyte ascorbic acid levels fall and remain low for up to 56 days. The vitamin C status stays low even with a normal diet containing 50 mg of ascorbate a day. A controlled trial has shown 4 grams of vitamin C per day raises the leucocyte vitamin C concentration quickly. These reports suggest myocardial infarct patients have poor ascorbic acid status and should be supplemented with vitamin C as soon after the event as possible.

Experiments have suggested two possible negative effects with large long term vitamin C supplementation. First, in a variety of laboratory animals, high doses of vitamin C impaired copper status and experimental copper deficiencies were exacerbated. These findings were extended to humans recently by Finley and Cerklewski. They supplemented 13 normal men at each meal with 500 mg vitamin C for 64 days, resulting in a continuing downtrend for serum copper and ceruloplasmin. The decrease was significant for ceruloplasmin. The copper and ceruloplasmin values rose after vitamin C supplementation was discontinued. These experiments suggest persons supplementing with large doses of vitamin C, say one gram or more per day, should make sure they are getting 2 mg of dietary copper per day.

A second possible problem is kidney stone formation due to increased oxalic acid excretion after vitamin C administration. The majority of persons have very moderate increases and are probably at low risk, but Briggs in 1973 found a small percentage of persons had enormous increases in oxalic acid excretion. Briggs work has not been confirmed by others. The latest work, including Schmidts in 1983, who used more reliable measuring tecniques, only found mild increases in urinary oxalate after massive (10 gram/day) doses of vitamin C. Overall, the majority of the evidence does not convincingly implicate vitamin C supplementation in kidney stone formation.

SUMMARY and RECOMMENDATIONS

Chronically low vitamin C status in animals produces many of the characteristics of human atherosclerosis. When poor vitamin C status is combined with dietary saturated fat and cholesterol, more advanced atherosclerosis results. Serum cholesterol and triglyceride are also elevated on low vitamin C regimens. Vitamin C supplements protect against rises in serum lipids and atherosclerosis from dietary lipids. Extensive human epidemiology supports a protective role for vitamin C. Clinical trials on patients have demonstrated vitamin C supplements reduce serum cholesterol and triglyceride. There is evidence heart attack patients have poor vitamin C status.

The evidence on vitamin C supports a diet higher in fruits and vegetables, which of course would crowd out calories from fat and sugar. This recommendation is consistent with the dietary advice given throughout this book.

The RDA for vitamin C is 60 mg. Most surveys report 30 to 50% of the population gets less than 45 mg per day. Ginter, a leading authority on vitamin C and CVD, suggests an RDA in the range of 200 to 300 mg would be preferable. If one examines the many fruits and vegetables which provide 60 mg or more per serving, it becomes obvious that the RDA is too easy to satisfy. This suggests the RDA may have been set too low.

The best sources for vitamin C are citrus fruits, berries, melons, tropical fruits, leafy green vegetables, broccoli, cauliflower, cabbage, green peppers, tomatoes, and potatoes. A one cup serving of most of these foods provides more than 100 mg of vitamin C. It reasonable to expect a good diet to contain a cup of vitamin C rich food with each meal. This would provide 300 to 400 mg of vitamin C daily.

REFERENCES

VITAMIN B6

Anonymous, Is vitamin B6 an antithrombogenic agent? Lancet 1:1299-1300,1981.

Anonymous, Inhibition of platelet aggregation and clotting by pyridoxal-5 phosphate. Nutr Rev 40:55-7,1982.

Boers, G. et. al. Heterozygosity for homocystinuria in premature peripheral vascular disease. NEJM 313:709-15,1985.

Chadefaux, B. et.al. Is absence of atheroma in Down Syndrome due to decreased homocysteine levels? Lancet 2:741,1988

Gruberg, E. & Raymond, S. Beyond Cholesterol. Vitamin B6, Arteriosclerosis and Your Heart. St. Martin's Press, New York, 1981.

Israelsson, B. et.al. Homocysteine & myocardial infarction Athero 71:227-33,1988

McCully, K. Homocysteine theory of arteriosclerosis: development and current status. Athero Rev 11:157-239,1983.

Mudd, S. Vascular Disease and Homocysteine Metabolism (editorial) N Eng J Med 313:751-3,1985.

Mulvaney, D. & Seronde, J. Electrocardiographic changes in vitamin B6 deficient rats. Cardiovas Res 13:506-13,1979.

Rinehart, J. and Greenberg, L. Vitamin B6 deficiency in the rhesus monkey with particular reference to the occurrence of atherosclerosis. Am J Clin Nutr 4:318-28,1956.

Rose, C. et. al. Age differences in vitamin B6 status of 617 men. Am J Clin Nutr 29:847-53,1976.

Rossouw, J. et. al. Lack of a relationship between plasma B-6 and IHD. S Afr Med J 67:539-41,1985.

Schoene, N., et. al. Effect of oral B-6 on in vitro platelet aggregation. Am J Clin Nutr 43:825-30,1986.

Serfontein, W. et. al. Plasma B-6 (PLP) level as risk index for CAD. Athero 55:357-61,1985.

Willett, W. Does low B-6 intake increase the risk of CHD? in Vitamin B-6:Its Role in Health and Disease, p337-46, Reynolds & Leklem, eds, 1985

VITAMIN C

Aulinskas, Ascorbate Increases the Number of LDL Receptors in Cultured Arterial Smooth Muscle. Athero 47:159-71,1983

Bordia, A. The effect of vitamin C on blood lipids, fibrinolytic activity and platelet adhesiveness in patients with coronary artery disease. Athero 35:181-7,1980.

Briggs, et. al. Urinary oxalate and vitamin C supplements. Lancet 2:201,1973.

Findley & Cerklewski.Influence of ascorbic acid supplements on copper status. Am J Clin Nutr 37:553-6,1983.

Ginter, E. Ascorbic Acid in Cholesterol and Bile Acid Metabolism. Ann NY Acad Sci 258:410-21,1975.

Ginter, E. Marginal Vitamin C Deficiency, Lipid Metabolism and Atherogenesis. Adv Lipid Res 16:167-220,1978.

Ginter, E. Pretreatment serum cholesterol and response to ascorbic acid. Lancet 2:958-9,1979.

Ginter, E. et. al. Vitamin C in atherosclerosis. Int J Vit Nutr Res Supp 19:55-70,1979.

Ginter and Bobek, The influence of Vitamin C on lipid metabolism. p.299-374. in Vitamin C, Counsell and Hornig, eds. Applied Science Publishers. 1981.

Heine, H and Norden, C. Vitamin C therapy in hyperlipoproteinemia. Int J Vit Nutr Res Supp 19:45-54,1979.

Horrobin, D. et. al. The Regulation of PGE-1 Formation: A candidate for one of the fundamental mechanisms involved in the actions of vitamin C. Med Hypoth 5:849-58,1979.

Schmidt, K. et. al. Urinary oxalate excretion after large intakes of ascorbic acid. Am J Clin Nutr 34:305-11,1981.

Sokoloff, B Effect of ascorbic acid on certain blood fat metabolism factors. J Nutr 91:107-18,1967.

Spittle, C. Vitamin C and deep vein thrombosis. Lancet 2:199-200,1973.

Sulkin, N & Sulkin, D. Tissue Changes Induced By Marginal Vitamin C Deficiency   Ann NY Acad Sci 258:317-28,1975.

Vallance, Hume and Weyers. Reassessment of changes in leucocyte and serum ascorbic acid after acute myocardial infarction.   Br Heart J   40:64-8,1978.

7. VITAMIN E and NIACIN

VITAMIN E

Vitamin E has been steeped in controversy since its discovery as a factor necessary for reproduction in female rats in 1922 by Evans and Bishop. In 1931 great excitement occured when it was shown vitamin E prevented nutritional muscular dystrophy in several laboratory animals. This excitement turned into confusion and disappointment when vitamin E administration produced no improvement in humans with muscular dystrophy. Adding to the confusion was the diverse variety of diseases produced in animals with vitamin E deficiency. Furthermore, some of the diseases could be prevented by nutrients other than vitamin E.

Human studies have also suffered from high hopes, confusion and contradictory results. Two recent excellent treatises on vitamin E make a point of noting the controversy surrounding vitamin E. Phillip Farrell from the University of Wisconsin wrote, " Despite over 50 years of intensive study and wide acceptance as an essential nutrient for lower animals, the status of vitamin E in human nutrition remains unsettled, if not enigmatic..... In fact, a comprehensive review of the literature on vitamin E in human health and disease conveys the strong impression that virtually all aspects of this nutrient's role in human beings are controversial." Milton Scott, in his outstanding chapter on vitamin E in the Handbook of Lipid Research, vol 2, writes "One group claims that vitamin E is the cure for almost every disease known to man; the other group takes the stand that vitamin E has not been proved scientifically to have any of the effects being claimed for it. The true value of vitamin E lies between these two extremes." It is important for readers to be aware of the diverse and extreme views held by many experts on vitamin E.

The oil soluble compounds having vitamin E activity were named tocopherols (tocos means childbirth and phero means to bring forth) by their discoverer Evans. There are numerous tocopherol isomers, the alpha, beta, gamma and delta forms are the most common. Alpha tocopherol has the greatest activity of them all.

Since vitamin E is oil soluble, its digestion and absorption is a function of the individual's ability to digest and absorb fat. Bile has been shown to be necessary for vitamin E absorption. Studies on humans using radioactive tocopherol reveal absorption rates of 50 to 86%. The major fraction is absorbed by the the lymphatic system and then dumped into the blood stream. Tocopherol is carried by various lipoproteins in the blood.

VITAMIN E DEFICIENCY

Vitamin E, along with selenium are antioxidants, both of which help prevent the oxidation of the polyunsaturated fat in cell membranes and cell organelles. Muscles and nerves have extensive membrane systems and are exposed to a continual flow of oxygen and hydrogen peroxide, making them susceptible to oxidative damage during vitamin E deficiency. We will see this is precisely where profound vitamin E deficiency symptoms occur.

Frank, severe deficiencies are rarely encountered in humans except in infants and patients with severely impaired fat absorption. For example, in abetalipoproteinemia, a rare inherited disease where fat and vitamin E are virtually unabsorbed, severe deficiencies of vitamin E result. Typically, serum levels of vitamin E are not detectable and devastating neurological and neuromuscular defects are produced after 10 or 20 years. Clinical trials lasting up to

15 years on children with abetalipoproteinemia using massive daily doses of vitamin E (2000 mg or more) have reported normal vitamin E levels in the supplemented patients along with normal neurological and neuromuscular function.

Other disorders of chronic fat and vitamin E malabsorption have reported severe neuromuscular dysfunction. Commonly low bile production and chronic liver disease are associated with impaired fat and vitamin E absorption. Trials with oral or intramuscular administration of vitamin E in these cases have resulted in improved neuromuscular function.

Patients with cystic fibrosis normally exhibit impaired vitamin E and fat absorption due to pancreatic dysfunction. Neuromuscular disorders, including heart muscle degeneration, are commonly reported with cystic fibrosis. Vitamin E supplements have reduced the symptoms of neuromuscular dysfunction in cystic fibrosis.

Autopsy studies of vitamin E deficient rats, monkeys and humans have revealed characteristic spinal column and peripheral nerve axon degeneration. An autopsy survey on cystic fibrosis demonstrated vitamin E supplementation had a strikingly beneficial effect on preventing nerve axon degeneration. There is little doubt severe, chronic vitamin E deficiencies result in neurological and neuromuscular degeneration and dysfunction.

Vitamin E deficiency is commonplace in premature infants due to a combination of poor tissue reserves, impaired absorption, low concentrations in formula milks and iron supplementation. Indeed, studies of premature infants have provided good support for vitamin E's essential role in human health. Full term infants also have low vitamin E values at birth, but these rapidly rise to normal in comparison to the chronic low values in premature infants.

Retinopathy of prematurity, usually called retrolental fibroplasia, was first reported in 1942. It is a major cause of impaired vision and blindness in childhood. Scar formation in the retinal blood vessels is the main cause of blindness in retrolental fibroplasia. The retinal vessels are not completed in premature infants. The normal growth of these vessels is adversely affected by high oxygen concentrations combined with low vitamin E levels. A number of controlled clinical trials using high doses of vitamin E have demon-

strated good results in preventing and limiting the severity
of retrolental fibroplasia. The latest double blind trial by
Hittner et. al. of 101 preterm infants reported excellent
results with high doses of vitamin E.

Vitamin E deficiency in cows, pigs, rats, mice, rabbits
and lambs also produces skeletal and heart muscle degeneration. The disease is characterized by muscle necrosis,
inflamation and replacement of the necrotic muscle tissue
with fat and fibrous tissue. There is progressive weakness
which correlates with the severity of the myopathy. In
addition, in the cardiovascular system there is arterial
necrosis with fibrous tissue replacement and calcification of
the cardiac lesions.

An interesting observation, reported many times in the
1940's and 1950's is vitamin E deficient muscle has a higher
rate of oxygen consumption. This could be of critical
importance during ischemic episodes in patients with coronary
artery disease. Ischemia with vitamin E deficiency would be
a scenario for an infarct, that is, reduced oxygen supply
coupled with increased oxygen demand.

More recently it was shown (Fujimoto) that vitamin E is
remarkably protective against cerebral ischemia in dogs. The
dogs were pretreated with vitamin E, then blood flow was
restricted to the brain for one hour, and then blood flow was
returned to normal (reperfusion). In the dogs without
vitamin E there was no recovery of brain electrical activity
but there was in the dogs pretreated with vitamin E. It is
thought by many workers that reperfusion after ischemia
produces a burst of peroxidation products and these lipid
peroxides cause a great deal of cellular damage. In this
study on dogs vitamin E very likely protected against the
reperfusion damage.

Some interesting animal work has been reported on vitamin
E with adriamycin, a cancer chemotheraputic drug. Adriamycin
in both animals and humans produces heart muscle degeneration
which appears similar to the heart muscle degeneration
occuring with vitamin E deficiency. Adriamycin causes
increased production of malonaldehyde, a lipid oxidation
product. Malonaldehyde is implicated in causing heart muscle
degeneration. Vitamin E administration during adriamycin
therapy greatly reduces malonaldehyde production and reduces
heart muscle degeneration in animals.

Chickens made vitamin E deficient develop a capillary degeneration known as exudative diathesis. Capillaries become very leaky and fluids flow from the capillaries into the tissue spaces. Exudative diathesis is not found in other animals, nor is atherosclerosis produced in animals with vitamin E deficiency.

PLATELETS and PROSTAGLANDINS

Many published studies have reported inhibition of platelet aggregation by vitamin E. Steiner in 1978 showed, with both in vitro and in vivo work, vitamin E inhibits platelet aggregation. The inhibition was dose dependent in human volunteers supplementing with 1200 to 2400 IU of vitamin E per day and also in vitro. When challenged with ADP, collagen or epinephrine (all of which cause platelets to aggregate), platelets from vitamin E supplemented subjects were inhibited 30 to 50%. When challenged with arachidonic acid (the polyunsaturated fat which is the direct precursor for the production of the aggregating prostaglandin thromboxane A-2) the platelets from vitamin E supplemented subjects were completely inhibited.

Karpen et. al. confirmed several previous reports of vitamin E's inhibition of platelet aggregation in the rat. They and others extended this intriging effect on platelets to an investigation of vitamin E's effects on prostaglandin synthesis. The results are extremely exciting, finally putting vitamin E therapy of cardiovascular disease on a rational basis. Karpen et. al. found higher thromboxane A-2 (TXA-2, the aggregating "bad" prostaglandin) production in platelets from vitamin E deficient rats. In addition, arterial tissue from vitamin E deficient rats produced markedly less prostacyclin (PGI-2, the powerful antiaggregating "good" prostaglandin made by endothelium). Vitamin E supplements reversed the situation by inhibiting TXA-2 production and raising arterial PGI-2 synthesis. A report on humans showed vitamin E supplements (1600 IU per day for seven days) increased prostacyclin production and decreased thromboxane synthesis in healthy volunteers. These are extremely important effects and they have been confirmed in other animal experiments.

Karpen et. al. studied human insulin dependent diabetics and non-diabetic controls, finding platelet TXA-2 production was inversely related to platelet vitamin E status, that is, with high platelet vitamin E there was low TXA-2 synthesis and vice versa. As a group, the 16 diabetics had significantly lower platelet vitamin E than matched controls and significantly higher TXA-2 production. This helps to explain the common finding of increased platelet aggregation in diabetics.

A landmark study on chemically (streptozotocin) induced diabetic rats by Karpen et. al. strongly supports the work on human diabetics. In this experiment there were three groups of animals: controls rats; diabetic rats; and diabetic rats supplemented with vitamin E. Inexplicably, the diabetic rats had greatly depleted platelet levels of vitamin E compared to control rats. Vitamin E supplements restored the diabetic rats platelet vitamin E values to above the control rats.

The diabetic rats, as expected because of their low platelet vitamin E concentrations, had sharply elevated TXA-2 production and reduced PGI-2 production. Vitamin E supplements in the diabetic animals increased the PGI-2 levels and reduced the TXA-2 concentrations in the diabetic animals. These experiments have important implications for the etiolology and treatment of diabetic vascular pathology. A clinical trial in 1955 on 41 diabetics claiming vitamin E supplements (400 to 600 IU per day) greatly improved their vascular lesions and ulcers now seems logical in light of Karpen's work.

A recent double blinded experiment from France (Colette) on nine type I (insulin dependent) diabetics using 1000 mg vitamin E for 35 days confirmed the previous work on animals. In the patients after vitamin E supplementation there was reduced platelet aggregation and less TXA-2 produced.

TREATMENT OF CVD

In a previous chapter we saw prostaglandin therapy had remarkable results on peripheral vascular disease patients. Many trials using vitamin E on peripheral vascular disease report significant benefit also. It seems reasonable to suggest vitamin E's effect on prostaglandin production is one of the reasons for the favorable outcomes.

When discussing the topic of vitamin E treatment of car-diovascular disease, it is critical to distinguish between treatment of coronary heart disease and peripheral vascular disease. With CHD there is great controversy and consid-erable doubt concerning vitamin E's efficacy, but with peripheral vascular disease, vitamin E therapy shows a consistent pattern of favorable results. An interesting parallel can be found with prostaglandin therapy: there is little consistent evidence it is effective for CHD, but substantial data shows it works for peripheral vascular disease. Three excellent reviews on vitamin E therapy for CVD are: Scott, Farrell and Marks.

PERIPHERAL VASCULAR DISEASE

Vitamin E supplements for intermittent claudication have been investigated for many years. In 1949 a trial with 76 patients showed 78% improvement after 6 months on vitamin E. In 1958 a double blind study on 34 patients lasting 10 months reported objective improvement. In 1963 Boyd and Marks did a controlled experiment for 3 months and the advanced patients on vitamin E demonstrated significant improvement over con-trols. Boyd and Marks also compared the survival rates of 1476 patients on vitamin E therapy with nine other published reports on longevity of intermittent claudication patients. They claimed a much higher survival rate for the vitamin E treated patients.

Haeger published a controlled trial on intermittent claudication in 1974 using blood flow to the extremities as the criteria for improvement rather than exercise tolerance. After 20 to 25 months of vitamin E therapy, there was almost a 40% average increase in blood flow to the lower legs in the vitamin E treated group compared to a 20% decrease in the control group. In addition, there have been several other reports claiming benefit with vitamin E therapy.

Haeger and others who have had extensive experience with vitamin E treatment of intermittent claudication, point out positive effects are usually not exhibited before three months of therapy. Secondly, daily doses between 300 and 600 IU appear to be effective, but below 200 IU there is little evidence of benefit.

There have been several trials reported as failures but in every case they either failed to give adequate amounts of vitamin E or didn't extend the treatment beyond three months. The scholarly reviewers give the postive trials more credence than the failures. In summary, we can say there is evidence, both theoretical and clinical, that long term vitamin E therapy benefits intermittent claudication.

A similar conclusion, but based on fewer trials, can be made for thrombophlebitis. Haeger, for example, reported controlled observations on 227 men with peripheral occlusive arterial disease. They were observed for two to five years. In the tocopherol group 9 patients died vs 19 in the control group. There was one limb amputation of a vitamin E patient but eleven amutations of non E patients. There was also a significant increase in exercise tolerance in the vitamin E group. Similarly, there are several reports on vitamin E reducing thromboembolism in surgical patients. The mechanism of action in both thrombophlebitis and thromboembolism is probably vitamin E's effect on platelet aggregation and the prostaglandins.

CARDIAC DISEASE

Vogelsang and Shute, of the Shute Clinic in Canada, first reported megadose supplements of vitamin E produced dramatic improvement in ischemic heart disease patients. The clinic continues to claim vitamin E benefits angina and other symptoms of coronary heart disease. The Shute Clinic has had more experience with vitamin E than any other group, having treated over 30,000 coronary heart disease patients.

Unfortunately the Shute Clinic does not do controlled studies, so most physicians are hesitant to use the results as a basis for their practice. Further, there have been at least 17 reports by other researchers who have not found vitamin E beneficial for CHD. Many of the reports were carefully controlled double blinded experiments. Some of the negative reports can be criticized for their small size and short duration. Nevertheless there are very few favorable studies on heart disease except from the Shute Clinic.

Toone in 1973 published one of the few double blind experiments showing positive results with vitamin E, but there were only 22 patients in the trial. All the subjects (angina patients) quit smoking, walked, lost weight and half of them were put on 1600 IU vitamin E per day for two years. At the end of the experiment there was a remarkable decrease in angina and nitroglycerine intake in the vitamin E group compared to controls.

The case for or against vitamin E therapy in cardiac disease has yet to be proved. The attitude towards vitamin E in the 1980's is different than in the 1970's due to the discoveries of the beneficial effect vitamin E has on prostaglandin production and platelet aggregation. There are now sophisticated and well accepted reasons why vitamin E should work, the question is, does it work? To see if vitamin E benefits CHD, a long term (at least two years, three or four years would be better), controlled trial with a large number of high risk subjects enrolled should be performed.

Another reason for renewed interest in vitamin E is its possible effect on HDL levels. Hermann et. al. in 1979 published a brief uncontrolled experiment on 10 persons, giving them 600 IU vitamin E per day for 40 days along with measuring the serum HDL levels. The serum HDL cholesterol was raised 375% in subjects with low initial values and 168% in subjects with normal initial values. Subsequent, better controlled experiments showed more modest increases in HDL cholesterol and the increases were only significant in those with low initial values.

There have been several studies confirming and several refuting Hermann's results on HDL levels. Herman has analysed the conflicting data and pointed out vitamin E only appears to increase HDL cholesterol in 1. subjects under 35 years of age. 2. subjects with low initial HDL cholesterol. 3. Subjects with elevated triglyceride and very low density lipoproteins and 4. response takes much longer in overweigh persons. According to Hermann's analysis, there is a substantial group of people in which HDL cholesterol can be raised by vitamin E administration. This is potentially a very useful finding.

ATHEROSCLEROSIS

Animals on vitamin E deficient regimens have not been reported to develop atherosclerosis at a higher rate than controls. Nevertheless there is some very interesting experimental and theoretical work on atherosclerosis implicating vitamin E as a protective factor.

The new work deals with the relationship between leucocytes (macrophages, monocytes and neutrophils), which are part of the immune system, and atherosclerosis. It has recently been discovered that foam cells, which are lipid filled and found in both fatty streaks and advanced fibrous plaque, are actually macrophages (white blood cells that scavenge bacteria and cellular debris).

There are many possible mechanisms whereby macrophages and other leucocytes could be involved in the development of atherosclerosis. One very clear way is through lipid infiltration. Macrophages in diseased arteries become engorged with lipids by ingesting LDL. The macrophages fill with fat and cholesterol until they burst, indicating the ingestion of LDL is unregulated. The dying, fat filled foam cells dump there contents into the arterial lesion, forming an important part of the "gruel" found in diseased arteries.

Macrophages only ingest 'altered' LDL and the alteration necessary appears to be the peroxidation of the LDL. Many cells and substances can peroxidize the lipids in LDL, including white blood cells (monocytes and neutrophils). Furthermore, peroxidized LDL has been shown to be cytotoxic, but non-oxidized LDL is not. Cathcart reported that vitamin E prevents the peroxidation of LDL by white blood cells. This could prove to be a landmark discovery.

Evidence on humans has now begun to appear. Lemoyne has demonstrated there is a sharp drop in lipid peroxidation in humans when they supplement with vitamin E. He used breath pentane to meausure the amount of lipid peroxidation. Stringer found significantly higher amounts of lipid peroxides in the plasma of persons with atherosclerosis. Gey et. al. reported lower plasma vitamin E in areas of Europe and Great Britain with high rates of CHD.

SUMMARY and RECOMMENDATIONS

Vitamin E deficient animals have heart and vascular pathology, greater production of "bad" prostaglandins, and increased platelet aggregation. Vitamin E supplements in animals and humans result in higher production of "good" prostaglandins, raised levels of the beneficial high density lipoproteins (HDL) and stabilized platelets. Long term benefit was reported for peripheral vascular disease patients using 200 to 600 IU vitamin E. The evidence on heart disease patients using vitamin E is inconsistent. Vitamin E is protective against cerebral ischemia in dogs. There is a great deal of new experimental work suggesting vitamin E could well be protective against the development of athero-sclerosis.

The recommendations for vitamin E rich diets are not consistent with the other recommendations made in this book, because high fat foods contain the most vitamin E. The RDA for vitamin E is 15 IU. It is difficult to obtain 15 IU per day on a low fat diet. Here are some vitamin E values for some representative foods:

Mayonnaise	2 tablespoons	30 IU
Corn oil	2 tablesppons	30
Cooked spinach	1/2 cup	2
Broccoli	1/2 cup	1
Whole wheat bread	2 slices	1
White bread	2 slices	0.1
Ground beef	3 ounces	0.6
Cornflakes	2 ounces	0.3
Tomato	1 medium	0.8

The above numbers indicate low fat diets usually provide less than 15 IU. Another aspect of vitamin E enters here, which is, the higher the fat intake, especially polyunsaturated fat, the greater the need for vitamin E. This means the requirement for vitamin E goes down on low fat diets.

The dosage of vitamin E used in therapuetic clinical trials is 30 to 50 times the amount you can get in a good, non oily diet. It is not possible to get this much by diet, whether it is oily or non oily. Thus we have the problem, should supplements be taken since you cannot get anything approaching a theraputic dose from food?

If one has peripheral vascular disease, the risk-reward ratio would seem favorable. What are the risks of supplementing with 200 to 600 IU daily for years? Even though vitamin E is an oil soluble vitamin, it has low toxicity. The Food and Nutrition Board of the National Research Council in 1980 stated 400 to 1000 IU daily did not produce adverse effects for most adults. Since the clinical trials used 200 to 600 IU with beneficial results, it seems foolish to go beyond those amounts.

Should coronary artery disease patients supplement? The risk-reward ratio is not as favorable, because most of the controlled clinical trials have not shown benefit. Nevertheless, other risk factors such as platelet aggregation and prostaglandin production have improved with vitamin E supplements. The extremely large amounts Dr. Shute uses (1500 to 3000 IU) have greater risk of side effects. In the absence of controlled trials at these high levels, it would seem prudent to stay within the 200 to 600 IU range. The reader should be aware the case for supplementing with vitamin E for coronary artery disease is not very strong because almost all of the controlled trials have been failures. Nevertheless the animal work showing protection against ischemia with vitamin E is very provocative. The experiments on lipid peroxidation and macrophages suggest the future for vitamin E with heart disease could be somewhat brighter.

Should healthy, symptom free persons supplement to prevent peripheral vascular disease? In this case the risk- reward ratio appears less favorable. The risk stays the same but there are no experiments to indicate how big the reward will be. With the new advances in lipid peroxidation, LDL and macrophages, it could well be future research will demonstrate a reward with vitamin E, but of course we will have to wait and let the future be the judge of that. If a sypmtom free person is supplementing, it is safer to be at the 200 IU range than the 600 IU range.

NIACIN

Nicotinic acid and nicotinamide are two forms of a vitamin called niacin. Pellegra, a potentially fatal niacin deficiency disease, is characterized by profound skin and gastrointestinal tract lesions and nervous system dysfunction which usually progresses to insanity. Niacin's RDA is 14 to 18 mg per day with as little as 10 mg daily preventing pellegra. In 1955 it was discovered that 3000 mg (3grams) of nicotinic acid per day reduces serum cholesterol and triglycerides in humans. Numerous studies have confirmed the initial findings. For example, in 1972 a nicotinic acid trial on 160 hyperlipidemic patients produced a 26% average reduction in serum cholesterol. Grundy et. al. in 1981 reported a 22% reduction in cholesterol and a 52% decrease in triglycerides. The mammoth Coronary Drug Project, with 1100 coronary artery disease patients taking 3000 mg of nicotinic acid daily compared to 2800 placebo controls, demonstrated a 10% decrease in serum cholesterol and a 26% reduction in triglycerides.

These studies leave little doubt but massive doses of nicotinic acid reduce serum lipids in hyperlipidemics. Unfortunately, doses below 1000 mg do not influence serum lipids. This means diet has little to do with niacin's hypocholesterolemic effect, since it is not possible to approach 1000 mg per day of niacin from food. Animal protein is the best source of niacin, but even by eating 10 cans of water packed tuna, the highest niacin food of all, one would only get 200 mg. Eating this much protein for any length of time would be dangerous due to the increased burden on the kidneys. Based on this dietary analysis, one can not argue that elevated serum cholesterol is due to mega-dose niacin deficiencies, since it is not possible, nor has it ever been possible to get 1000 mg of niacin daily from food. Probably niacin at high doses acts like a drug and not like an essential nutrient.

Pharmacologic doses of niacin have additional beneficial effects. The protective high density lipoproteins (HDL) are raised and the atherogenic low density lipoproteins (LDL) are lowered. Reduced levels of non-esterified fatty acids have also been reported in controled trials. Other documented effects are increased fibrinolytic activity (clot disolving activity), increased platelet stability and vasodilation. These remarkable properties are probably due to nicotinic acid's stimulation of PGI-2 and PGE-1 production, both of which are beneficial prostaglandins. It was discussed in a previous chapter that PGI-2, given intravenously, can reverse atherosclerosis in advanced peripheral vascular disease. Both PGI-2 and PGE-1 stabilize platelets, increase fibrinolytic activity and dilate arterioles. In addition nicotinic acid inhibits the production of TXA-2 by platelets. TXA-2 contracts arterioles and increases platelet aggregation, hence the inhibition of this 'bad' prostaglandin by niacin is another important pharmacological effect.

The above factors are probably the reasons high doses of nicotinic acid inhibits atherosclerosis in animals fed atherogenic diets. Further, the 29% reduction in non-fatal myocardial infarctions experienced by the nicotinic acid group in the Coronary Drug Project (1100 subjects and 2800 controls) now appears very reasonable in light of nicotinic acids multifacedted actions.

Since 1986 there has been a steady stream of glowing reports on niacin therapy. A fifteen year mortality study of the Coronary Drug Project showed niacin lowered the death rate from all causes, including cardiovascular disease, 11%. The other medications in this massive study (estrogen, clofibrate, and dextrothyroxine) were no better than placebo. This remarkable result for niacin has never been demonstrated for any other cholesterol lowering substance, including cholestyramine (indeed in the Lipid Research Clinics Program using cholestyramine lowered heart disease death rate but not death from all causes).

Blankenhorn et. al. reported Colestipol-niacin therapy after 2 years lowered LDL by 43%, raised HDL by 37%, significantly slowed or stopped coronary artery athero-sclerosis in the majority of patients and regressed atherosclerosis in 16% of the patients. Cohen and Morgan also reported remarkable long term benefits, including regression of atherosclerosis, in patients with niacin or niacin with Probucol. Malloy et. al., using a combination of Lovastatin, Colestipol and niacin on patients with severe hypercholesterolemia, produced serum cholesterol reductions averaging 55%. The addition of niacin to the regimen was of great benefit. The medical establishment now considers niacin an important lipid lowering drug, alone or in combination with other drugs.

There are side effects with massive doses even though niacin is a water soluble vitamin with extremely low toxicity (the LD-50 for rats is 5 to 7g/kg, which on a weight adjusted basis is 350g for a 70kg human). The most common side effect is the 'niacin flush', a rather intense feeling of heat and reddening of the skin, usually occuring on the upper body and face. The flush can occur at doses of 50mg and commonly is reduced in intensity after repeated doses. There is no evidence the 'niacin flush' is harmful or symtomatic of bodily harm, but it is a nuisance.

A more important adverse effect is impaired oral glucose tolerance. This impairment could be due to the liver releasing more glycogen to compensate for the decreased levels of non-esterified fatty acids. Persons with diabetes mellitus should be given megadose niacin cautiously. Higher uric acid values is another important but less common side effect. Patients with gout, of course, should be closely monitored. Also, it should be pointed out, most subjects experience a rebound elevation of serum lipids after discontinuing megadose niacin.

DOSE and BLOOD LEVELS

A one gram dose produces a 200 to 1000 fold increase in plasma niacin levels after one hour and then falls rapidly. To counteract the rapid fall, most experimental protocols specify three doses per day. Another strategy is the manufacture of slow releasing analogues of nicotinic acid. There has been good sucess in reducing the dosage using these analogues. One common niacin derivative, niacinamide does not produce the 'niacin flush', but unfortunately it does not lower serum lipids.

SUMMARY and RECOMMENDATIONS

Improved diets will not provide enough nicotinic acid to lower blood lipids or improve prostaglandin production. Hence the question on niacin is, should one take megadose supplements? Obviously if you have normal serum lipids, the answer is no. With elevated lipid levels, diet should be tried first and this book provides much information on that strategy. If lipids remain high in the face of pronounced dietary change, then it is a question of what medication, if any, to take. Niacin at one to three grams per day should be considered a drug. It is a cheap drug, quite safe and has powerfully benefical effects on prostaglandins, serum lipids, lipoproteins, platelets, atherosclerosis, heart attack rate, and death rate, but decisions on what drug to take are best made between patient and doctor.

REFERENCES

VITAMIN E

Barboriak, J. et.al. Vitamin E and Plasma High Density Lipoprotein Cholesterol. Am J Clin Path 77:371-2,1982.

Cathcart, M. et al. Monocytes and neutrophils oxidize LDL making it cytotoxic. J Leuko Biol 38:341-50,1985.

Colette, C. et.al. Platelet function in type I diabetes: effect of Vitamin E. Am J Clin Nutr 47:256-61,1988.

Chan, A. and Leith, M. Decreased PGI-2 Synthesis in Vitamin E deficient Rabbit Aorta. Am J Clin Nutr 34:2341-7,1981.

Fitzgerald, G. & Brash, A. Endogenous PGI-2 and TXA-2 During Vitamin E Therapy. Ann NY Acad Sci 393:209-1,1982.

Fujimoto, S. et.al. Protective effect of vitamin E on cerebral ischemia. Surg Neurol 22:449-54,1984.

Gey, K. et. al. Plasma levels of antioxidant vitamins in relation to IHD & Cancer Am J Clin Nutr 45:1368-77,1987.

Gillilan,R.et.al. Evaluation of Vitamin E in the Treatment of Angina Pectoris. Am Heart J 93:444-9,1977.

Haeger,K. Long-term observation of patients with athero-sclerotic dysbasia on Vitamin E. in Tocopherol, Oxygen and Biomembranes. deDuve and Hayaishi eds. 1977, pp 329-332.

Hermann,W. The Effect of Vitamin E on Lipoprotein Cholesterol Distribution. Ann NY Acad Sci 393:467-72,1982.

Horwitt, M. Supplementation with vitamin E. Am J Clin Nutr 47:1088,1988 (letter)

Karpen, C. et.al. Restoration of Prostacyclin/Thromboxane Balance in the Diabetic Rat. Diabetes 31:947-51,1982.

Karpen, C. et.al. Platelet Vitamin E and TXA-2 Synthesis in Type I Diabetes Mellitus. Diabetes 33:239-43,1984.

Lemoyne, M. et.al. Breath pentane analysis:index of lipid peroxidation & vitamin E. Am J Clin Nutr 46:267-72,1987

Mitchinson,M & Ball, R. Macrophages and Atherogenesis. Lancet 2:146-9,1987.

Muller, D. et.al. Vitamin E and neurological function. Lancet 1:225-8,1983.

Nelson, J. Pathology of vitamin E Deficiency. in Vitamin E: A Comprehensive Treatise. Machlin, ed. 1980, pp 397-427.

Olson,R. Vitamin E and Its Relation to Heart Disease. Circ 48:179-84,1973.

Scott, M. Vitamin E in Handbook of Lipid Research, vol 2, 1978, DeLuca, ed. pp. 133-210.

Steiner, M. Inhibition of platelet aggregation by vitamin E in Tocopherol, Oxygen and Biomembranes. deDuve and Hayaishi eds. 1977, pp 143-164.

Stringer, M. et.al. Lipid Peroxides and atherosclerosis. Br Med J 298:281-4,1989.

Sundaram, G. Alpha-tocopherol & serum lipoproteins. Lipids 16:223-7,1981.

NIACIN

Blankenhorn, D. et. al. Beneficial effects of Colestipol-niacin Therapy on Coronary Atherosclerosis and Coronary Bypass Grafts.   J Am Med Assn 257:3233-40,1987

Canner, P. et.al. 15 year mortality in Coronary Drug Project Patients: Niacin. J Am Coll Cardio 8:1245-55,1986

Carlson, L. et. al. Reduction of MI with clofibrate and nicotinic acid.   Athero 24:81-6,1977

Cohen, L. & Morgan J.   Niacin and Probucol in reduction of serum cholesterol. J Fam Pract   26:145-50,1988

Grundy, S. et. al.Nicotinic acid and metabolism of choles-terol and TG in man.   J Lipid Res 22:24-36,1981

Gurian & Aldersberg. Effect of large doses of niacin on lipids and carbo. tolerance. Am J Med Sci 237:12-22,1959.

Holz, W., Niacin and its derivatives.   Adv Lipid Res 20: 195-217,1983.

Malloy, M. et. al. Colestipol, Niacin and Lovastatin in treatment of severe familial hypercholesterolemia   Ann Int Med 107:616-23,1987.

Parsons, W.   Treatment of hypercholesterolemia by nicotinic acid.   Arch Intern Med 107:639-52,1961.

Walldius, G. & Wahlberg, G.   Effects of nicotinic acid and its derivatives on lipid metabolism and other factors. Adv Exp Med Biol 183:281-94,1985.

8. VITAMIN D, TRANS FAT and LECITHIN

VITAMIN D

Vitamin D is more properly classified as a steroid hormone than a vitamin. It is made from cholesterol by skin exposed to sunlight. If skin is exposed to adequate sunlight, there is no dietary requirement for vitamin D. Except for eggs, lard, butter and fish liver oils, few foods contain vitamin D. Supplemental vitamin D is added to milk, margarine, cereals, bakery goods and breakfast drinks.

Excessive vitamin D produces blood vessel pathology, a fact which has been know since 1928. Most recently, Taura et. al. induced coronary atherosclerosis in pigs using excessive vitamin D for three months along with a low fat, low cholesterol diet of corn and soybean meal. These animals had normal serum cholesterol and no dietary stresses except excess vitamin D. The control animals had no lesions or abnormal areas in their arteries. Swine sacrificed immediately after three months of vitamin D feeding had calcification of the internal elastic membrane and thickened intima with excessive smooth muscle and connective tissue. Animals sacrificed three months after the vitamin D feeding had classic atherosclerosis in the left decending coronary artery, which is the most common and lethal location of

atherosclerosis in humans.   The atherosclerotic lesions
occured above the calcified internal elastic membrane. The
lesions, found in all the vitamin D treated animals, contained fat and cholesterol deposits, necrotic tissue, raised
thickened intima, and excessive connective tissue.   These
results are sobering.   They illustrate the devastating effect
excessive vitamin D can have on arteries.

The standard protocol for producing atherosclerosis in
dogs, rats, and mice calls for excessive vitamin D along
with fat and cholesterol.   Cattle, horses and rabbits also
exhibit vascular lesions in response to vitamin D rich diets.
Furthermore, excess vitamin D causes diminished magnesium
status.

HUMAN WORK

The epidemic of coronary artery disease in Western countries parallels the introduction and increased use of vitamin
D in infant formulas, milk, cereals and vitamin pills.   Prior
to 1920 the primary source of vitamin D was skin exposed to
sunlight.   The RDA for children is 400 IU and adults is
200 IU.   Many surveys report a large percentage of children
and adults ingest two or more times the RDA.

The risks of excessive vitamin D during infancy are well
documented. In Germany and Great Britain outbreaks of infant
hypercalcemia, artery and heart valve lesions (supravalvular
aortic stenosis syndrome) with mental retardation was closely
associated with vitamin D consumption and treatment.   Many
papers and reviews have brought forth evidence on the tragic
consequences of excessive vitamin D in infants.   A survey in
Canada in 1972 reported 70% of the children under 5 years of
age consumed more than 400 IU per day and 30% more than
1000 IU daily.   Rickets can be prevented with 100 IU of
vitamin D per day.

Linden in 1977 investigated the vitamin D consumption of
118 myocardial infarct patients and 118 age matched controls.
He found infarct patients were ingesting an average of 50%
more vitamin D than the healthy controls.   The patients
averaged 1200 IU per day, six times the RDA.   Analysis of the
data showed an intake above 1200 IU daily was closely associated with increased risk of myocardial infarct.

Vitamin D is one of the few vitamins Americans commonly get in excessive amounts. It is also the one with the smallest margin of safety. The RDA is 400 IU for children, whereas 100 IU prevents rickets. The primary reason for fortifying foods and nutrient supplements with vitamin D is to prevent rickets. The RDA for adults is 200 IU. A survey of young adults in 1967 reported 50% took 400 to 800 IU daily and 10% more than 1000 IU a day.

SUMMARY and RECOMMENDATIONS: VITAMIN D

Excess vitamin D has been utilized as a promoter, in conjunction with fat and cholesterol, of atherosclerosis in animals. Recently, vitamin D produced atherosclerosis in the coronary arteries of pigs without any other dietary stresses. These are important findings.

Certain types of arterial and heart valve pathology in infants are closely associated with excess vitamin D. Historically, there is a disturbing parallel between the rapid rise of vitamin D supplementation and the epidemic of coronary artery disease in the Western world. A survey of infarct patients in Norway found their average vitamin D intake to be 6 times higher than the RDA and significantly higher than age matched controls. Many surveys show the majority of infants, children and adults consume two or more times the RDA.

The evidence discussed here does not constitute 'proof' that excess vitamin D is responsible for a good percentage of our CVD, but it is disturbing enough to persuade a prudent person to severely limit their intake of vitamin D. In terms of risk-reward ratios, there are no rewards but many risks when taking excessive vitamin D.

Supplements are the biggest problem with vitamin D. Almost all multivitamin supplements contain 400 IU per tablet. There are many special supplements containing even more vitamin D, such as, fish liver oil capsules, cod liver oil, calcium supplements and A&D capsules. Many persons easily obtain 1200 IU per day from supplements. Do not supplement with more than 400 IU per day.

Milk contains 400 IU per quart, but buttermilk and yogurt do not contain added vitamin D. Most cold cereals have 40 IU per ounce (8 years ago many had 400 IU per ounce). Some bakery goods and breakfast beverages contain 50 IU per serving. One supplement along with one quart of milk and five ounces of cold cereal sums to 1000 IU of vitamin D. Read labels. Try to stay at or below 400 IU per day.

TRANS FAT

Naturally occuring unsaturated fatty acids are normally in the cis geometric configuration. During the process of partial hydrogenation, many of the cis fats are flipped into the trans geometrical form. Trans fatty acids are considered unsaturated for labeling purposes, but they have a higher melting point than cis acids so they help margarines remain solid at room temperature. The figure below shows the relationship between cis and trans molecules:

C-C   C-C   partial   C-C
   \   /   --------------------->   \
    C=C   hydrogenation   C=C
                                                 \
                                                  C-C

cis   trans

Except for small amounts of trans fat in cow's milk all other naturally occuring fatty acids are cis. The consumption of trans fat has increased markedly in the United States because margarines and many salad oils contain partially hydrogenated oils. A number of reports reveal margarines are rich in trans fat. The Institute of Shortening and Edible Oils reports the majority of partially hydrogenated liquid oils contain 10 to 25% trans fat and solid hydrogenated frying fats usually range from 5 to 25% trans. Most stick margarines are 20 to 35% trans.

The amount of trans fat may be of interest because some experiments suggest it may contribute to the development of vascular disease and alter various physiological properties of cells. As with almost all fat research, there are a number of conflicting reports and opinions on the trans fat problem.

ANIMAL STUDIES

Trans fat, when fed to rats, is absorbed at the same rate as cis fat. It is deposited in tissues and the amount found there is directly related to dietary intake. For example, rats fed a diet containing 10% of the calories from trans rich margarine, had 17% trans fat in the carcass. When half the margarine was replaced with olive oil, there was only 10% trans fat in the carcass. After two months on a trans free diet, the trans content of the carcass was reduced to 3%.

Both cis and trans fat are used for energy by cells at the same rate. There are some studies which show trans fat depresses the conversion rate of linoleic acid to arachidonic acid, the precursor of many prostaglandins. In addition, there is a considerable slowing down in the speed at which trans fat attaches itself to cholesterol and breaks apart from cholesterol. Also, polyunsaturated trans fat does not act as an essential fatty acid and it can not be used to make prostaglandins.

Since fat, especially unsaturated fat, forms a major part of cell membrane, it is not surprising to find trans fat in cell membranes. One study reported trans fat is incorporated into brain cell membranes of immature and mature rats. Possible long term subtle effects could occur here.

Decker and Mertz published a report demonstrating under some conditions trans fat in membranes can alter the permiability and stability of the membrane significantly. Red blood cells with incorporated trans fat burst five times more rapidly in the presence of the enzyme lecithinase than red blood cells without trans fat. Mitochondria from rats fed trans fat swelled 2 to 3 times faster in hypotonic solution than those from control rats. This indicated the trans fat altered the permiability of the membrane but there were a number of experimental conditions where the cis and trans membranes behaved almost identically.

Rats fed purified trans fat exhibited higher serum cholesterol than controls. Rabbits fed trans fat and cholesterol had higher serum cholesterol and more atherosclerosis than rabbits fed olive oil with cholesterol. Recently Kritchevsky fed trans fat without added cholesterol to rabbits observing significant increases in serum cholesterol and triglycerides but no increase in atherosclerosis. He fed the the same diet to vervet monkeys without increased atherosclerosis or blood lipids.

Kummerow et. al reported swine fed trans fat for 8 months developed raised vascular lesions compared to almost no blood vessel pathology in animals given butterfat or beef tallow. These results were criticized because the animals may have had essential fatty acid deficiency. The experiments were repeated making sure they had sufficient essential fatty acids. Kummerow did not find elevated serum lipids or atherosclerosis in the new trials with adequate essential fatty acids. All of the recent results suggest trans fats are not damaging to arteries.

HUMAN WORK

The amount of trans fat found in human milk was reported to be a function of the mothers consumption of trans fat. This suggests, when combined with animal experiments, infants nursed by mothers on high trans diets will have trans fat incorporated into the cell membranes of the central nervous system. The consequences of this are unknown.

Vergroesen claimed trans fat increased serum cholesterol in human subjects when compared to controls on cis fat. Anderson also found higher serum cholesterol in subjects consuming trans fat. Kummerow pointed out the diets in the National Heart Study contained different amounts of trans fat. The serum cholesterol in each group appeared to be a direct function of trans fat content of the diet. He also showed the amount of trans fat found in red blood cells correlates with CHD death rates in Finland, Bulgaria, Romania and the United States.

In an experiment on 33 adult males, Mattson et. al. did not find serum cholesterol was a function of trans fat. Meyer, from the Institute of Shortening and Edible Oils also gathered evidence which suggests trans fat does not raise serum cholesterol. Human studies, it appears, have given conflicting results.

SUMMARY and RECOMMENDATIONS: TRANS FAT

Animal work mildly suggests trans fat may, to a small extent, promote CVD. Trans fats do not have essential fatty acid activity and they may inhibit prostaglandin production. The fact it does alter some cell membrane characteristics and it is incorporated into nervous tissue, even during infancy, means it could have long term subtle effects on humans. The direct evidence on trans fat and human CVD is sketchy and conflicting.

Since there is no evidence showing trans fats are beneficial and some evidence they are mildly harmful, it would seem prudent to avoid excessive consumption of trans fat. Furthermore, persons on low fat diets run the risk of developing essential fatty acid deficiency and impaired prostaglandin production if the limited fat they consume is mostly trans fat. Persons on low lipid diets would be wise to rely on nuts, seeds or oils which are rich in polyunsaturated fats and low in trans fat.

Excessive trans fat consumption can be avoided by limiting consumption of partially hydrogenated fats and oils. This means reducing the use of margarine, soybean oil and cotton seed oil, all of which are partially hydrogenated. Corn, sunflower seed, safflower, olive and walnut oils are not partially hydrogenated, hence these oils do not contain trans fat. Nuts and seeds do not contain trans fat either. Walnuts are interesting, since they contain more essential fatty acids than any other nut or seed. Three walnuts daily will prevent essential fatty acid deficiency.

LECITHIN

Lecithin is a popular supplement with many vague claims for its ability to "fight cholesterol." Everybody seems to "know" lecithin is an emulsifier which dissolves blood lipids, rendering them harmless. Let us examine this concept more carefully. It is true, lecithin is an emulsifier which helps, in conjunction with protein, to dissolve lipids. Almost all the lipids are carried in the blood as lipoproteins, a series of blood soluble complexes containing fat, protein, cholesterol, and lecithin. Nevertheless, the safety or harmfulness of lipids does not depend on their solubility. The atherogenicity of lipids depends on the type and amount of lipoprotein it is incorporated in. Low density lipoproteins, for example, are harmful when elevated even though the lipids are soluble, but high density lipoproteins are beneficial, especially when elevated. The claim that lecithin makes lipids safe by dissolving them is completely false. This is a situation where knowing a few facts is a dangerous thing, because it leads to completely unwarranted and untrue conclusions on lecithin's effects.

Lecithin is derived from a fat molecule. Fat, more properly called a triglyceride, is composed of three fatty acids connected to a glycerol molecule. Lecithin has two fatty acids instead of three. The third is replaced by a phosphate choline group. Lecithin's emulsifying property is due to the phosphate-choline group. Lecithin can be synthesized by the liver if choline is available. The key to lecithin production is choline, since the liver can make all the lecithin needed if there is enough choline.

Choline is required in the diet by some animal species. It is not known if humans have a dietary choline requirement, since the liver can produce it if there is sufficient folic acid, methionine, and vitamin B-12 available. Except for fruits and vegetables, choline is found in a wide variety of foods as part of the lecithin molecule. The average choline intake has been estimated to be 400 to 900 mg per day. Three grams of pure lecithin supplies over 400 mg of choline. Recently there has been interest in choline supplements for Alzheimer's disease because it is a precursor to the neurotransmitter acetylcholine. The results using choline on advanced stage Alzheimer's disease are not encouraging.

ANIMAL WORK: LECITHIN

Intravenous administration of choline or lecithin produces strikingly beneficial effects on the cardiovascular system but oral treatment does not. For example, intravenous choline lowers blood pressure in both animals and humans but equivalent oral doses do not. The effect of intravenous and oral lecithin on blood pressure has not been reported for animals or humans.

Rabbits, when put on high cholesterol diets for 3 to 4 months usually develop cholesterol laden atherosclerotic lesions. There are now many experiments showing significant regression of these cholesterol induced lesions in rabbits if they are given several intravenous infusions of lecithin after the cholesterol feeding. It did not appear to matter whether the lecithin is from soybean or brain. In rats with dietary induced atherosclerosis, intravenous lecithin decreased the size and extent of the vascular lesions. Minipigs had regression of atherosclerosis with intravenous lecithin. In quail, intravenous lecithin dramatically reduced arterial lesions.

Studies with baboons have additional importance because of the similarity to human metabolism. In one experiment, baboons had severe atherosclerosis induced by six months of dietary abuse and 12 injections of bovine serum albumin. The baboons given 3 weekly injections of one gram of lecithin had greatly reduced atherosclerosis.

We can see intravenous lecithin is remarkably effective in regressing experimentally induced atherosclerosis in a wide variety of animals. It is important to note there are differences between experimentally produced lesions in animals and naturally occuring fibrous plaque in humans. The difference in induction time helps to illustrate this. Experimental lesions take three to six months to develop, but human atherosclerosis usually requires 15 to 40 years.

In sharp contrast to the excellent results with intravenous administration, oral lecithin has produced conflicting results. There have been few oral animal experiments published, possibly because none of them had positive results to report. Some of the animal work shows serum cholesterol is raised after oral lecithin administration. Almost all of the human lecithin work has been with oral treatment and very few intravenous experiments. Indeed, it is a curious situation to have the human trials follow the path of the least promising animal experiments and ignore the exciting leads from the intravenous animal work.

HUMAN WORK: LECITHIN

The trials on humans have almost exclusively been oral treatments with conflicting results. Daily doses of one to two grams of soy lecithin per day have not affected serum cholesterol or triglyceride in hyperlipidemics or normals. On the other hand, extremely high amounts of lecithin, up to 48 grams per day, have lowered serum lipid levels. Since lecithin is 76% fat, 48 grams of lecithin provides 36 grams of fat, most of it polyunsaturated. For comparison, one third cube of butter or margarine contains 36 grams of fat and 325 calories. The average lecithin capsule weighs 1.2 grams, so it would take 40 capsules to equal 48 grams of lecithin. I think you can see doses in the range of 30 to 50 grams are very large, high calorie, and would be a great nuisance if taken in capsule form.

Tompkins and Parkin did an uncontrolled trial on five persons using 48 grams of soy lecithin for 2 years and reported an average 16% decrease in serum cholesterol. This trial not only had few subjects and no controls, but the subjects received 36 grams of salad oil via the lecithin. It is well known that salad oils moderately lower serum cholesterol by themselves.

Morrison in 1958 reported dramatic (41%) serum cholesterol decreases in 12 hypercholesterolemic patients put on 36 grams of granular lecithin per day, but there were important flaws in this experiment. First, there were no controls. Second, 21 patients started, 6 dropped out due to side effects, 3 didn't respond and one patient had an unbelievable serum cholesterol reduction from 1012 mg% to 186 mg%. If the 3 non responders are included and the bizzare fall from 1012 to 186 is eliminated, then the net reduction was 19% and not 41%, but we still have the problem of how to evaluate the 6 drop outs. Third, the supplement was not all lecithin. It was 29% lecithin, 29% cephalin and 32% inositol phosphatides. Fourth, the polyunsaturated fat content of the supplement could account for a large part of the 19% decline in serum cholesterol. Frankly, there are too many flaws in Morrison's experiment to be able to use the results in a meaningful way.

Three reports (Greten, 1979; Childs, 1977; and Simons, 1977) using 20 to 40 grams of soy lecithin demonstrate lecithin's cholesterol lowering effect is due to its poly-unsaturated fat content. All three studies gave lecithin or an equivalent amount of corn or soy oil to subjects. The serum cholesterol response was the same for both lecithin or the equivalent amount of salad oil. These controlled trials provide good evidence that lecithin's hypocholesterolemic property, when given in massive doses is due to its large polyunsaturated fat content.

To date, Blaton et. al. have done the only intravenous lecithin experiment on humans. They gave one gram of lecithin intravenously per day for 14 days to 93 patients with elevated serum lipids. After 14 days there was a 10 to 12% average drop in serum cholesterol. This study does demonstrate intravenous lecithin is much more effective than oral, but it misses the point of the animal work, which showed intravenous lecithin regressed experimental atherosclerosis. It is completely impractical to lower serum cholesterol by intravenous administration due to the great cost and considerable risk. Work needs to be done on humans to see if intravenous lecithin regresses human atherosclerosis, because the reward in this case would be more than worth the risk and cost.

SUMMARY and RECOMMENDATIONS: LECITHIN

Intravenous lecithin regresses experimental atherosclerosis in animals, but no meaningful intravenous work has been done on humans. Oral administration of 1 to 2 grams daily to humans does not lower serum cholesterol. Massive doses, in the range of 20 to 50 grams, do lower serum cholesterol, but the effect has been shown to be very likely due to the salad oil content of the lecithin and not the lecithin. Massive doses are not practical long term (or short term for that matter) because of the high fat, high calorie content (up to 350 calories per day), high cost and gastrointestinal side effects of the lecithin. Experimental evidence does not support supplementation with lecithin for CVD prevention or treatment.

REFERENCES

VITAMIN D

Kent, S. et. al. Hypervitaminosis D in monkeys. Am J Path 34:37-59,1958.

Kummerow, F. Nutrition imbalance and angiotoxins as dietary risk factors in CHD. Am J Clin Nutr 32:58-83,1979

Linden, Correlation of vitamin D intake to IHD, Hypercholesterolemia, & Renal Calcinosis. in Nutritional Imbalances in Infant and Adult Disease. Seelig, ed. 1977 SP Books.

Seelig, M. Magnesium Deficiency in the Pathogenesis of Disease. Plenum Medical Book Co. 1980

Taura, S. et. al. Vitamin D-induced coronary atherosclerosis in normolipemic swine. Tohoku J Exp Med 129:9-16,1979.

TRANS FAT

Cook. H. The influence of trans acids on desaturation and elongation of fatty acids in developing brain. Lipids 16: 921-926,1981

Decker, W. and Mertz, W. Effects of dietary elaidic acid on membrane function in rat mitochondria and erythrocytes. J Nutr 91:324-30,1967.

Kritchevsky, D. Trans fatty acid effects in experimental atherosclerosis. Fed Proc 41:2813-7,1982.

Kummerow, F. et. al. The influence of 3 sources of dietary fats and cholesterol on lipid composition of swine serum lipids and aorta tissue. Artery 4:360-384,1978.

Kummerow, F. Letter, Am J Clin Nutr 34:601-2,1981.

Kummerow, F. Current studies on relation of fat to health. J Am Oil Chem Soc 51:255-9,1974.

Royce, S. et. al. The influence of dietary isomeric and saturated fatty acids on atherosclerosis and eicosanoid synthesis in swine. Am J Clin Nutr 39:215-22,1984.

Sgoutas,D. and Kummerow,F. Incorporation of trans fatty acids into tissue lipids. Am J Clin Nutr 23:1111-9,1970

LECITHIN

Blaton, V. et. al. Effect of polyunsaturated phosphatidylcholine on human types II and IV hyperlipoproteinemia. Artery 2:309-25,1976.

Childs, M. et. al. Dietary lecithin vs corn oil. Clinical Research 25:159A,1977

Greten, H. et. al. The effect of polyunsaturated phophatidylcholine on plasma lipids and fecal sterol excretion. Athero 32:141,1979.

Morrison, L. Serum cholesterol reduction with lecithin. Geriatrics 12-19,1958.

Simons, L., et. al. Treatment of hypercholesterolaemia with oral lecithin. Aust NZ J Med 7:262-6,1977.

Sirtori, C., Phospholipids, atherosclerosis and aging in Phospholipids and Atherosclerosis. Avogaro et.al.editors Raven Press N.Y. 1983

Tompkins, R. and Parkin, L. Effects of long-term ingestion of soya phospholipids on serum lipids in humans. Am J Surg 140:360-4,1980.

Zeisel, S, Dietary Choline:Biochemistry, Physiology, and Pharmacology. Ann Rev Nutr 1:95-121,1981.

9. PROTEIN, CARBOHYDRATE and FIBER

PROTEIN

A neglected component of diet which influences serum cholesterol and atherosclerosis in both animal and human experiments is protein. The lack of interest in proteins influence on CVD risk factors is a paradox because the first successful dietary induction of atherosclerosis in animals was accomplished in 1908 using animal protein. A few years later it was demonstrated atherosclerosis could be induced in rabbits by using cholesterol. The previous experiments were reinterpreted, blaming the cholesterol in the diet and ignoring animal protein as a possible causative factor. From 1913 until the mid 1960's, there was astonishingly little interest in protein even though several experiments showed animal protein could cause atherosclerosis without added cholesterol.

ANIMAL STUDIES

Protein's relationship to atherosclerosis in laboratory animals is variable, depending on other dietary components. Rabbits have been studied more systematically and thoroughly than any other animal. The serum cholesterol of rabbits varies dramatically, depending on the type of protein included in the diet. Animal protein, primarily casein, skim milk, lactalbumin, extracted egg and beef protein elevated serum cholesterol the most, while raw egg white and pork protein only raised it moderately. Wheat gluten and peanut protein did not change serum cholesterol compared to controls but soy protein concentrate and soy protein isolate reduced it precipitously after 28 days. The hypercholesterolemic effects of beef or casein were eliminated by adding soy protein.

The type of protein not only effects serum cholesterol, but it also influences the development of atherosclerosis Dogs, monkeys and rabbits given casein or other animal proteins which raise serum cholesterol develop atherosclerotic lesions. The opposite is true with plant proteins. They keep serum cholesterol low and do not promote atherosclerosis. The addition of soy protein to casein or beef protein inhibits the development of atherosclerosis. In these experiments none of the diets contained cholesterol.

The reason for the marked difference between animal and vegetable protein on atherosclerosis and serum cholesterol is not fully understood. One problem is that pure protein is difficult to obtain. In general the protein preparations, whether animal or vegetable, contain very little fat, but do contain 30 to 40% non-protein material. Even casein and isolated soy protein contain 5 to 10% non-protein molecules. It is possible the non-protein material is influencing serum cholesterol and development of atherosclerosis, but this possibility has not been investigated.

When pure amino acid mixtures, identical to those found in casein, are fed to animals serum cholesterol is elevated as much as with casein. On the other hand, an amino acid mixture corresponding to soy protein produces higher serum cholesterol than soy protein. Amino acids added to casein producing an amino acid content similar to soy protein do not significantly lower serum cholesterol. Similar confounding results were found when amino acids were added to soy protein, giving it the amino acid content of casein. The added amino acids did not raise serum cholesterol.

David Kritchevsky, one of the leaders in protein and atherosclerosis research, has evidence the size of the lysine

arginine ratio in the protein affects the amount of atherosclerosis produced. There are other reports claiming exactly
the opposite of Kritchevsky's lysine/arginine results. K.K.
Carroll, another major leader in this field, has not been
able to confirm any of the results on the lysine-arginine
ratio. The effects of amino acids appear to be complex and
unpredictable. The consensus of the reviewers on this
subject maintain the amino acid content of the protein is
part of the protein-serum cholesterol riddle, but as you can
see from the inconsistencies cited here, it is not the whole
story.

We have more variables to face. For example, the type of
carbohydrate influences the animal versus vegetable protein
response. Casein plus glucose results in high serum cholesterol, but if raw potatoe starch is substituted for the
glucose, then added casein does not raise the serum cholesterol. Rice starch produced a similar effect and wheat
starch influenced soy protein but not casein. Cellulose,
the standard fiber used in animal experiments, when combined
with casein, raises serum cholesterol and when combined with
soy protein, lowers the cholesterol. If wheat straw is used
instead of cellulose, cholesterol levels are't changed, but
the atherogenicity of casein is reduced. When alfalfa
replaces cellulose, serum cholesterol and atherogenicity are
reduced and indistinguishable for both casein and soy protein. Alfalfa's ability to eliminate the adverse effects of
casein is remarkable.

There are a number of experiments showing polyunsaturated
fats can also eliminate the negative effects of casein and
other animal proteins. Protein interacts with dietary
constituents in a complex and poorly understood fashion.
Nevertheless, the animal experiments provide convincing
evidence that the type of protein is an important variable
for serum cholesterol and atherosclerosis.

HUMAN WORK

The epidemiology on protein supports but by no means
proves protein has a role in human CVD. All of the epidemiological studies have the problem of confounding variables,
that is, people or populations who primarily consume vege-

table protein usually eat more fiber, starch, and PUFA and less cholesterol, simple sugars and saturated fat. This same criticism can be leveled at the epidemiology of fat, sugar or fiber. All of them have the unresolvable problem of intermingled variables. With this caution in mind, we can point out numerous studies demonstrating vegetarians have significantly lower serum cholesterol, triglycerides and CHD mortality than matched non-vegetarian controls. Internationally, there is a strong correlation between a nation's animal protein consumption and coronary heart disease mortality. Historically, the rise of animal protein consumption combined with the decline in vegetable protein intake fits quite well with the rise in CHD mortality in the U.S. This is in sharp contrast to the lack of any historical relationship between saturated fat or cholesterol consumption and CHD mortality in the U.S.

Clinical trials for the most part have shown protein type influences risk factors, some of them strikingly so. Carroll et. al. reported moderate but significant reduction of serum cholesterol when soy protein was substituted for animal protein in healthy young women. This well controlled study held dietary fat, cholesterol and carbohydrate almost constant for both the animal and vegetable protein diets. This was not a low fat trial, since 40% of the calories came from fat. Van Raaij et. al. studied the effects of soy protein and casein on serum lipoprotein and cholesterol levels in 69 healthy subjects. The average serum cholesterol did not change, but on the soy protein diet there was a significant rise in beneficial serum HDL and a fall in atherogenic LDL.

Sirtori et. al. in two well controlled experiments, reported remarkable declines in serum LDL and cholesterol when textured soy protein isolate (Temptein-Miles Labs) was substituted for animal protein on a low fat regimen. The subjects had stable type II hyperlipoproteinaemia with very high serum cholesterol, averaging about 350 mg%. All of the subjects had been on low fat-low cholesterol diets for three months prior with no noticible effect. In the first experiment, after three weeks on the soy diet, there was a 21% drop in serum cholesterol and in the second study there was an impressive 24% fall in cholesterol in 127 subjects after 8 weeks. This remarkable reduction of serum cholesterol was maintained by replacing animal protein with soy protein in only one meal each day.

Verillo et. al. extended the findings on soy protein to sixteen weeks. In a study of 57 hyperlipidemic patients they found that adding 60 grams of textured soy protein to the diet worked as well as replacing the animal protein with the textured soy protein. Serum cholesterol was lowered an amazing 30% and LDL reduced 36%.

The authors of these reports emphasize these were low fat, low cholesterol regimens with a PUFA to saturated fat ratio of around two. They point out the soy protein works best in conjunction with a low fat regimen and on subjects with significantly elevated serum cholesterol (above 300). Surprisingly, the amount of cholesterol in the diet didn't seem to matter. During one part of a trial 500 mg of cholesterol was added and the soy protein continued to lower the serum cholesterol.

SUMMARY and RECOMMENDATIONS: PROTEIN

We have seen a number of lines of evidence suggesting vegetable protein offers protection against CVD and animal protein promotes CVD. The case is not closed. More evidence is needed and maybe future research will not support our conclusions here. Nevertheless, switching from animal protein to vegetable protein has many other lines of research supporting it. By eating more vegetable protein, you would be getting more fiber, complex carbohydrates, potassium, PUFA, copper, magnesium, and selenium and less cholesterol, saturated fat, and sodium. The results on protein provides another supporting link in our dietary argument.

SUGAR

Yudkin first reported a relationship between a nation's sucrose consumption and CVD in 1957. He proposed sucrose could be as much of a risk factor as fat. Lopez in 1966 showed a significant relationship with sugar and serum cholesterol in 16 nations. On the other hand, prospective studies on people living within one country or area usually do not find a link between sugar and CVD. For example, the Framingham Study found no correlation for sugar and CVD. The large Puerto Rico (8218 subjects) and Honolulu (7272 persons) surveys did not report a correlation with sugar either. Both fat and sugar appear to have similar problems with inconsistent epidemiology. This is reasonable since sucrose and fat consumption are highly correlated both nationally and internationally.

Animal work suggests sucrose may play a role in atherosclerosis. Serum cholesterol is elevated in rats put on high sucrose diets. In rabbits and baboons, arterial pathology is greater with sucrose rich diets. The sucrose work on animals is not as extensive or persuasive as the animal experiments using fat.

There has been limited human experimentation. Yudkin reports about 30% of his subjects respond to high sucrose diets with increased platelet aggregation. He also found a greater percentage of CVD patients have this abnormal response to sucrose than healthy controls. Trials measuring the effect of sucrose on serum cholesterol have produced conflicting results. Some showed no effect and others using 30% sucrose had elevations in serum cholesterol and triglyceride. An interesting discovery was made when glucose was substituted for sucrose. After four weeks on glucose, serum cholesterol fell 30% in a trial with 18 subjects. No prevention trials have been done using sucrose as a variable.

COMPLEX CARBOHYDRATES

Cereals, grains, potatoes, flours, legumes and vegetables contain "complex" carbohydrates. Complex carbohydrates contain the digestible polysaccharide starch and indigestible fiber polysaccharides such as cellulose, pectin, gums and lignin.

Internationally, epidemiology supports a protective role for complex carbohydrates. Generally those countries with greater complex carbohydrate consumption have fewer CVD deaths. A 16 nation study also revealed reduced serum cholesterol with greater intake of these substances. An important prospective study in London found these food components appeared to protect against CVD.

The ten year Zutphen Study reported CHD death rate was four times higher in persons consuming the least amount of complex carbohydrates. The large Honolulu and Puerto Rico prospective surveys found persons who developed CHD ate less of these food factors. There is more consistent epidemiology supporting complex carbohydrates as protective factors than there is implicating saturated fat and cholesterol as harmful agents.

A curious and common finding in diet surveys is persons who develop CHD consume <u>fewer</u> calories than persons free of CHD. In other words, calories appear to be protective. Little difference is seen in fat and sugar ingestion, leaving complex carbohydrates as the variable behind the differing caloric intakes. Persons consuming more calories with less CHD in general are eating more complex carbohydrates.

The data on calories being protective does not mean obesity is beneficial. In fact obesity is a well documented risk factor. These findings were on a weigh adjusted basis. The secret to eating more calories and maintaining normal weight is exercise. The statistics on calories being protective is also support for exercise as a protective factor.

Animal work is consistent with the human epidemiology. Starch, fiber and vegetable protein (found in foods with complex carbohydrates) in general lower serum cholesterol and inhibit the development of atherosclerosis in laboratory animals.

SUMMARY and RECOMMENDATIONS:
SUGAR and CARBOHYDRATES

The epidemiology, although not uniform, on balance implicates sucrose as a risk factor. Limited animal work and human trials support sucrose as a moderate promoter of CHD.

Complex carbohydrates have the opposite relationship. There is substantial epidemiology linking complex carbohydrates with protection against CHD. The epidemiology for this protective factor is stronger than for saturated fat and cholesterol as causes of CVD. The animal work is supportive of a protective role for complex carbohydrates.

This is another link in our dietary argument. The recommendations based on this data are in agreement with other recommendations in this book, namely, avoid promoters of CVD and increase protective factors. Avoiding fat and sugar leaves more room for complex carbohydrates. They are protective and also contain more fiber and nutrients than fat and sugar. Vegetables, potatoes, legumes and whole grains are the best sources of complex carbohydrates.

FIBER

Fiber was popularized in the United States by the publication in 1975 of David Reuben's book, The Save Your Life Diet. Reuben overstated the case for fiber and indeed trivialized the nature of cardiovascular disease. In 1982 the best selling high fiber book, The F Plan Diet, attests to fibers continued popularity and public appeal. Before 1969 there was little professional or public interest in roughage even though Walker and Arvidsson in 1954 and T.L. Cleave a few years later begin publishing evidence that low fiber diets may be an important cause of Western degenerative diseases. In 1969 Burkitt published a landmark paper in The Lancet which galvanized professional interest in fiber.

The primary molecules that plants synthesize are simple sugars, such as glucose or fructose, which they link together to form sugar polymers or polysaccharides. Some of the polysaccharides, primarily starches, are digestable, but most of the polysaccharides are refractive to human digestive enzymes.

Dietary fiber is defined as the indigestable polysaccharides or carbohydrates. There are many different classes of fiber molecules, for example, cellulose, hemicelluloses, lignins, pectins, gums and mucilages and they have widely differing properities. Some of the fiber molecules are not "digested" even when they are first boiled with sulfuric acid and subsequently boiled with sodium hydroxide. These resistant molecules are called crude fiber. It is beyond the intended scope of this book to discuss the various fiber molecules in detail. An excellent set of reviews and critical papers on fiber's role in health, including gastrointestinal disorders, cancer, diabetes, obesity and cardiovascular disease can be found in the October 1978 supplement of the American Journal of Clinical Nutrition.

EPIDEMIOLOGY: FIBER

The first convincing evidence put forward supporting fiber's protection against cardiovascular disease was based on epidemiology of African tribes. A number of English physicians pointed out the rarity of cardiovascular disease, especially coronary artery disease in black African tribes. They also noticed the absence of other Western degenerative diseases like diabetes, cancer of the colon, diverticular disease, and obesity and reasoned it would be difficult to claim low fat intake was the main protective factor for all of these diseases. Further, there were areas in Africa where fat consumption had been growing for many years and CVD was still low there. The English physicians concluded the African's high roughage diet was a significant protective factor.

Fiber rich diets in general are low in fat and the obverse is generally true, that is, fiber poor diets tend to be high in fat. Repeated and extensive dietary surveys, both national and international, have established that animal fat, vegetable fat, sugar, complex carbohydrates, animal protein, vegetable protein and fiber are not independent variables. This means low fat countries are invariably low in sugar and animal protein, but rich in fiber and complex carbohydrates. The opposite is true for high fat countries. Certainly it is extremely difficult, using epidemiology alone, to prove one factor is the most important and the others are insignificant.

Experimental animal and human evidence is needed to make any claims based on epidemiology believable. There is animal and some human evidence to support the saturated fat case, but there is also experimental evidence to support fiber, animal protein, vegetable protein, sugar and complex carbohydrates as factors in CVD. What can you do in the the face of these seemingly contradictory results? If a person is looking for the one dietary cause of CVD, then I think you face a hopeless task. On the other hand, if you realize there is no a priori reason why there should only be one dietary cause of CVD and not many causes, then it makes it easier to deal intelligently with the evidence on fat, sugar, fiber, protein and so on.

There is additional epidemiological evidence on fiber. Western man, since the turn of the century has been eating less bread and potatoes, which is an important source of roughage. The bread that is eaten has less fiber in it now than at the turn of the century. A major difference between 19th century and 20th century diets is our reduced fiber intake, which fits with our tremendous increase in CVD in the 20th century. In the section on fat we pointed out fat intake has changed little in the United States since the end of the 19th century. Other studies show Italian-Americans consume more roughage and have half the ischemic heart disease mortality of comparable Americans on similar high fat diets.

Reports on vegetarian groups in the United States reveals an inverse relationship between dietary fiber and serum cholesterol. An international study of 16 non-affluent countries demonstrated a remarkably high inverse correlation between serum cholesterol and complex carbohydrate consumption, even though all of these countries had low fat diets. On another track, Trowell reported an extremely close parallel between ischemic heart disease and diverticular disease death rates in English women from 1930 to 1970. A similar parallel was reported for pulmonary embolism and diverticular disease in women. Diverticular disease is, for the most part, caused by inadequate dietary fiber. In summary there is strong epidemiological evidence supporting fiber as a protective factor against CVD.

ANIMAL EXPERIMENTS

Many experiments report serum cholesterol reductions with various added fibers. A few noticible exceptions stand out. Cellulose and bran, for example, do not lower serum cholesterol in animals. Pectin, on the other hand, found in most fruits and some vegetables, consistently lowers serum cholesterol in rats, chickens and rabbits. Starch from corn, rice or potato reduce serum cholesterol in the rat. Guar gum and carageenan depresses serum cholesterol in a variety of animals. Alfalfa and leguminous seeds lower serum cholesterol in rats and rabbits. Ground corn, barley, and oats reduce serum levels in rabbits and chickens.

In the late 1950's it was found saturated fat without cho- lesterol could occasionally cause atherosclerosis in rabbits. Later Kritchevsky discovered the atherosclerosis induced by saturated fat occured on fiber free regimens and did not occur when fiber was included. Since then many experiments demonstrate fiber inhibits experimental atherosclerosis. Monkeys, baboons, chickens, rats and rabbits have developed less atherosclerosis when they are supplemented with fiber, except for cellulose. Thus, fiber appears to be an important protective factor against experimental atherosclerosis in animals.

HUMAN STUDIES

A recent 10 year prospective study on 871 middle aged men reported strikingly lower coronary heart disease death rates in those consuming high fiber diets compared to men with low fiber regimens. Further, there was no difference in saturated fat consumption between the high and low death rate groups. Death from CHD was 4 times higher in the low fiber group compared to the high fiber group and death from all causes was 3 times higher. Another prospective study on 337 middle aged men also reported lower CHD death rates in the high fiber group. In addition vegetarians have lower serum cholesterol than non-vegetarians, on average about 28% lower than comparable persons in the same country. Vegetarians, of course, consume copious amounts of fiber.

Extensive studies on wheat bran, the supplement advocated by David Reuben (The Save Your Life Diet) to prevent CVD, conclusively show that wheat bran does not lower serum cholesterol. Wheat bran primarily contains water insoluble fiber and water insoluble fiber does not lower serum choles- terol in either animals or humans. The principal water insoluble fibers are cellulose, lignin and some hemicell- uloses. These fibers increase fecal bulk, delay glucose absorption, accellerate the rate food goes through the intestines, but do not lower serum cholesterol. Most grains and many vegetables contain water insoluble fiber.

The important water soluble fibers are pectin, gums, starch and some hemicelluloses. Barley, fruits, oats, especially oat bran, and dried beans are the main sources of water soluble fiber. Soluble fiber slows the rate food passes through the intestines, retards glucose absorption and significantly <u>lowers</u> serum cholesterol in animals and humans. Two factors are thought to be involved in the cholesterol reduction: 1. Soluble fiber binds with bile acids, impairing their reabsorption and use by the liver. Bile acids are reprocessed in the liver to make lipoproteins such as LDL cholesterol. 2. Soluble fiber is fermented in the colon into short chain fatty acids such as butyric, acetic and proprionic acid. These fatty acids very likely inhibit the livers ability to synthesize cholesterol and increase the body's ability to remove LDL cholesterol. Also of interest is butyric acids documented anti-carcinogenic properties.

As early as the 1950's Ancel Keys demonstrated that beans lowered serum lipids in humans. In the 1960's and 1970's many human trials were published on guar gum, pectin, beans and oats revealing serum cholesterol reductions in the range of 10% to 32%. These remarkable reductions slowly began to impress the establishment, especially when it became painfully apparent that the American Heart Association's low cholesterol, low saturated fat diet only lowered serum cholesterol by 5% to 7% and did even less for serum triglyceride.

In 1984 Anderson began publishing his marvelous results with hyperlipidemic patients put on water soluble fiber supplements, namely oat bran and beans. Now, five years later, Post Cereals, Kelloggs, and Quaker Oats are battling it out for market share of the oat bran cold cereal market. Recently the price of unprocessed oat bran in bulk doubled to $1.69/lb, further testimony to oat brans sudden but belated popularity. Let's look at the clinical results fueling this current popularity.

An initial study on diabetic men using about six ounces of oat bran added to a very low fat diet (12% fat) produced a 32% reduction in serum cholesterol after three weeks. Another study of 37 diabetic men concluded after 3 weeks with serum cholesterol 25% lower. Using three ounces of oat bran or dried beans on 20 hypercholesterolemic men decreased serum cholesterol by 19% after three weeks. Other studies followed similar men on oat bran or beans for 99 weeks with average serum cholesterol 22% lower, LDL cholesterol 29% lower and HDL cholesterol raised by 9%. When oat bran was added to typical high fat, high cholesterol diets serum cholesterol was reduced 13% after three weeks.

Most of the experiments reported, in addition to being rich in soluble fiber, were also high in carbohydrate, ranging from 55% to 70% carbohydrate. Usually high carbohydrate diets raise triglyceride levels but high carbohydrate, high soluble fiber regimens lower serum triglyceride. Anderson has reported triglycerides reduced by 20 to 25% in normals using oat bran or beans. Twelve patients with elevated triglycerides (ave.= 1143mg TG/dl) after 10 days of soluble fiber achieved an average 63% reduction in serum triglyceride.

Anderson's general high fiber diet recommendation is: 1. 55% or more calories from carbohydrates (two thirds or more from complex carbohydrates) 2. Protein should comprise 15% to 20% of calories, with a minimum of 45 grams of protein per day. 3. Less than 25% of calories from fat and less than 10% from saturated fat. 4. Less than 200 mg cholesterol. 5. More than 40 grams of total plant fiber.

The following is the total fiber (TF) and water soluble fiber (WSF) content in grams of 3.5 ounce servings of each food: Oat bran= 30g TF, 15g WSF. Rolled oats= 15g TF, 8.5g WSF. Wheat bran= 46g TF, 3.6g WSF. Corn Flakes= 13g TF 7.5g WSF. Grape Nuts= 14g TF, 6g WSF. Pinto beans cooked= 29g TF, 13g WSF. White beans cooked= 27g TF, 12g WSF. Kidney beans cooked= 29g TF, 13g WSF.

SUMMARY and RECOMMENDATIONS: FIBER

Countries and persons consuming high fiber diets have sharply lower CHD death rates than low fiber countries or persons. Animal studies show fiber, except for cellulose and wheat bran, reduces serum cholesterol and inhibits experimental atherosclerosis. Human clinical trials report water soluble fiber depresses serum cholesterol in normals and hyperlipidemics by a remarkable 19% to 32%. Triglycerides in normals are reduced 20% to 25%, but in hypertriglyceridemics it has been reduced an amazing 63%. These results merit the close attention of anyone interested in lowering serum lipid levels.

REFERENCES

PROTEIN

Carroll, K., Dietary protein in relation to plasma cholesterol levels and atherosclerosis.   Nutr Rev 36:1-5,1978

Carroll, K, Hypercholesterolemia & atherosclerosis: effects
of dietary protein. Fed Proc 41:2792-6,1982.

Carroll, K., et. al. Hypocholesterolemic effect of soybean
protein. Am J Clin Nutr 31:1312-21,1978.

Descovich, Sirtori, et. al.   Multicentre study of soybean
protein diet. Lancet 2:709-12,1980.

Kritchevsky, D., Vegetable protein and atherosclerosis.
J Am Oil Chem Soc 56:135-40,1979.

Sirtori, C. et. al. Soybean protein diet in the treatment of
type II hyperlipidemia. Lancet 1:275-7,1977.

Van Raaij, et. al. Effects of casein vs soy protein diets on
cholesterol & lipoproteins Am J Clin Nutr 34:1261-71,1981.

Verillo, A. et. al. Soybean Protein Diets in the Management
of Hyperlipoproteinaemia.   Athero 54:321-31,1985.

SUGAR and CARBOHYDRATES

Gordon, T. et. al. Diet and its relation to coronary heart
disease and death in 3 populations. Circ 63:500-15,1981

Kritchevsky, et.al. Influence of carbohydrate type on
atherosclerosis in baboons. Am J Clin Nutr 33:1869-87,1980

Kromhout, D. et. al. Dietary fibre and 10-year mortaltiy from
CHD, cancer and all causes. Lancet 2:518-21,1982.

Lopez, A. et.al. Some relationships between dietary carbohydrates & serum cholesterol. Am J Clin Nutr 18:149,1966

Story, J. Dietary carbohydrate and atherosclerosis. Fed Proc 41:2790-2800,1982.

Yudkin, J. Sweet and Dangerous, Bantam Books, New York, 1972

FIBER

Anderson,J & Bridges,S. Dietary fiber content of selected foods. Am J Clin Nutr 47:440-7,1988

Anderson, J. et. al. Hypocholesterolemic effects of oat-bran or bean intake. Am J Clin Nutr 40:1146-55,1984.

Anderson, J. & Gustafson, N. High-carbohydrate, high-fiber diet. Postgraduate Med 82(4):40-55,1987.

Heaton, K. et. al. Not just fibre-the consequences of refined carbohydrate foods. Human Nutr 37C:31- 35,1983.

Kritchevsky, D. Dietary Fiber. Ann Rev Nutr 8:301-28, 1988.

Kritchevsky, D. Fiber, lipids and atherosclerosis. Am J Clin Nutr 31:S65-S74,1978.

Kromhout, D., et. al. Dietary fibre and 10-year mortality from CHD and all causes. Lancet 2:518-22,1982

Podell, R. Feeling your oats and eating them too. Postgraduate Med 77(8):279-288,1985.

Trowell, H and Burkitt, D., Dietary fiber and cardiovascular disease. Artery 3:107-119,1977.

Tuomilehto, J. et. al. Long term treatment of severe hypercholesterolaemia with guar gum. Athero 72:157-162, 1988.

Vahouny, G., Dietary fiber, lipid metabolism, and atherosclerosis. Fed Proc 41:2801-6,1982.

10. MILK and ALCOHOL

MILK

Cow's milk has been accused of causing atherosclerosis for many years. There are two main theories for milk's alleged ability to promote arterial disease. The first is fairly obvious, that is, milk contains cholesterol (134 mg/qt) and saturated fat (23 g/qt =200 cal/qt), hence milk should elevate serum cholesterol and triglyceride by small but measurable amounts. Since serum cholesterol and triglyceride are well established risk factors, increases in these should promote vascular pathology.

The other theory of milk's alleged harmful properties deals specifically with homogenized milk. The homogenization process produces small fat droplets, possibly containing the enzyme xanthine oxidase. It was proposed the xanthine oxidase is absorbed unaltered with the fat droplets of homogenized milk and then the enzyme goes on to cause atherosclerosis. We will look at both theories individually.

MILK and SERUM LIPIDS

It seems reasonable to expect milk, containing saturated fat and cholesterol, to raise serum lipids in humans. Reasonable or not, milk, even extremely large quantities, does not raise serum cholesterol or triglyceride, but rather, quite unexpectedly, milk appears to reduce these risk factors.

Dr. George Mann first noticed this when he studied the Maasai tribe in Africa. The Maasai consume large quantities of milk and meat, yet they have a very low incidence of CVD and atherosclerosis. Mann did a controlled study of 24 Maasai men for 3 weeks, providing unlimited quantities of fermented whole milk and then measuring serum cholesterol. The milk consumption became enormous, averaging 8 liters (a little more than 2 gallons) a day. Many of them gained over 5 pounds in 3 weeks. The greatest surprise was the 9% fall in serum cholesterol. Another surprise was the men who gained more than 5 pounds had a much greater drop in serum cholesterol (19%) than the men who gained less than 5 pounds (6% fall). Weight gain is normally considered a cause of elevated cholesterol. Mann did another experiment using yogurt on 26 adults in the U.S. and confirmed the remarkable serum cholesterol reduction with 2 to 4 liters of whole or skim milk yogurt daily.

In 1977 Howard and Marks reported the results of adding two quarts of skim or whole milk to the regimen of 16 adults for two weeks. Serum cholesterol fell 5% in the whole milk group and 15% in the skim milk group. Howard and Marks confirmed the cholesterol lowering property of milk in a later publication. When one considers two quarts of whole milk contains 270 mg of cholesterol and 46 grams of saturated fat, it is indeed surprising a significant drop in serum levels occurs. The equivalent amount of butter (4 oz) found in two quarts of milk given daily to volunteers raised serum cholesterol by 15%.

Animal work has supported the human results. Experiments on rats have shown extracts of cow's milk inhibit cholesterol synthesis by the liver. Recent results have demonstrated there are two compounds present in human milk which inhibit cholesterol synthesis also. There is little question but milk, especially skim milk and yogurt made from skim milk, moderately lowers serum cholesterol. The mechanism is most likely the blocking of cholesterol synthesis by compounds found in milk. Clearly, the theory that cow's milk causes atherosclerosis by raising serum cholesterol is false. Milk lowers serum cholesterol, it does not raise it.

BOVINE MILK XANTHINE OXIDASE and ATHEROSCLEROSIS

This theory is more complex, so it is more important to deal with it because the theory sounds plausable and has many people frightened of drinking milk. Oster in a number of publications beginning in 1977 (see Clifford et. al. for references) proposed homogenized milk causes arterial depletion of a molecule similar to lecithin called plasmalogen. Oster's hypothesis is that xanthine oxidase, found in cow's milk, is absorbed by the intestinal tract unaltered from homogenized milk. Then the xanthine oxidase depletes the arterial plamalogen by an indirect process, thereby causing atherosclerosis. Clifford, in a recent review, collected evidence demonstrating Oster's theory is probably incorrect.

Let's examine the theory point by point. First, the case for arterial plasmalogen loss being a cause of atherosclerosis is extremely weak. There are a few early analyses showing arterial plasmalogen is depleted with age and atherosclerosis. These reports have been criticized due to inadequate controls, standards and reliable analytical tecniques for detecting plasmalogen. Even if there is plasmalogen loss during the development of atherosclerosis, it says nothing about causation of atherosclerosis. It would be similar to saying body wasting is the cause of malnutrition since wasting and malnutrition are highly correlated. There is no evidence supporting plasmalogen loss as a cause of atherosclerosis.

Second, the evidence for elevated bovine milk xanthine oxidase concentrations in atherosclerotic vascular tissue is tenuous. Very few direct analyses of arterial tissue have been done, but in the ones that have, there were no criteria for distinguishing normal from diseased arteries. Also, the method of analysis used could not differentiate between bovine xanthine oxidase and endogeneously produced xanthine oxidase. Measurements of xanthine oxidase in the serum have been plagued by the same problems, namely, the method of analysis used could not determine the source of the xanthine oxidase and control measurements were poorly selected.

Third, there is good evidence xanthine oxidase is not absorbed from the intestinal tract, regardless of whether its from homogenized cow's milk or any other source. Xanthine oxidase is inactivated in the stomach. In rats given milk or cream fortified with xanthine oxidase, no xanthine oxidase was detected in the lymph, indicating the enzyme was not absorbed from the GI tract. A number of other experiments on rats and pigs reported no xanthine oxidase absorbed from the GI tract either. Further, Ho and Clifford administered the enxyme directly into the arteries of rabbits and observed no depletion of arterial or cardiac plasmalogen, nor was there any evidence of plaque formation. Even if minute amounts of bovine xanthine oxidase were absorbed from the GI tract, one wonders how that would be a problem if large amounts given intravenously do not cause damage.

There is no palpable evidence homogenized milk is a major or even minor cause of CVD. Indeed, the experiments on serum cholesterol suggest milk is a protective factor, especially non-fat milk or yogurt. They are exceedingly high in calcium, providing about 300 mg per cup of milk and 400 mg per cup of yogurt. The section on hypertension and calcium links good calcium intakes with lower blood pressure, which is another finding in milk's favor.

Even though there are good reasons for drinking milk or eating yogurt, they are not sufficient to mimic the two to eight quart consumption rates of some of the clinical trials. Two to eight quarts provide too many calories, too much protein and calcium. This chapter was not written to rationalize huge intakes of milk, but rather to demonstrate milk is not harmful to the cardiovascular system and ordinary reasonable amounts are safe.

One well established problem with milk for some people is lactose intolerance. Milk contains lactose (milk sugar) and many adults lose the ability to digest lactose in the small intestine. This permits the lactose to move into the large intestine, providing sustenance for bacteria, usually resulting in flatulence, and sometimes diarrhea, inflamation and discomfort. In cases of lactose intolerance, yogurt is a good substitute because the lactose is predigested by bacteria during the production of yogurt.

SUMMARY and RECOMMENDATIONS: MILK

Even though whole milk contains saturated fat and cholesterol, it does not raise serum cholesterol or triglyceride.

In fact, there are now many reports demonstrating milk products, especially skim milk and yogurt, reduce serum cholesterol. A substance has been discovered in milk which inhibits cholesterol synthesis.

There is a theory that the enzyme xanthine oxidase from homogenized milk causes atherosclerosis. This theory has been shown to have no experimental or factual basis.

Milk is a good source of many nutrients, especially calcium. Recent epidemiology and experimentation suggests calcium protects against hypertension. Adults should be encouraged to consume skim milk or non fat yogurt. These products lower serum cholesterol, possibly protect against hypertension and supply many important nutrients.

ALCOHOL

A remarkable number of prospective studies have shown persons who consume moderate amounts of alcohol have a lower risk for developing cardiovascular disease, especially coronary heart disease. When you consider dietary saturated fat and cholesterol rarely show up as risk factors in prospective studies, it makes the data on alcohol seem more significant.

Gordon et. al. in 1981 summarized the results of three prospective surveys: the Framingham Study, the Honolulu Heart Study and the Puerto Rico Heart Health Program, containing 16,349 men ages 45 to 64. Comparing persons who subsequently developed coronary heart disease and those who did not, there were no differences in saturated fat or cholesterol intake, but there were differences in alcohol, starch and caloric intake. Persons who did not develop coronary heart disease had higher alcohol, starch and caloric intake. Alcohol, starch and calories appeared to protect against coronary heart disease.

Klatsky in 1974 found moderate alcohol consumption a protective factor in 464 subjects and so did the Boston Collaborative Study of 399 myocardial infarct cases and 2486 controls. Similar results were reported for a 11,000 man prospective study in Yugoslavia. Several additional reports have shown the same protective relationship between alcohol and coronary heart disease. Some notable exceptions are the

Western Electric Study and the Iowa Farmer Mortality report.
In the analysis of 62,000 male deaths in Iowa, farmers had
lower heart disease death rates than non-farmers, but farmers
had one half the alcohol intake of non-farmers.

The other exception is the Western Electric Study. It
found consumers of alcohol had a higher heart disease death
rate than non drinkers, but they were only looking at heavy
drinkers (more than 5 drinks per day). The study did not
evaluate moderate drinking, so the results are not in con-
flict with the majority of the other reports. The Western
Electric data on heavy drinking has been supported in most of
the other studies, that is, heavy drinking increases total
mortality and heart disease death rate.

The relationship between alcohol consumption and heart
disease death rate appears to be a U shaped curve, meaning
at low consumption there is a higher heart death rate, at
moderate intakes there is a lower death rate , but at high
consumption the heart death rate goes back up, forming a U
shaped graph.

Another aspect of some of the prospective studies should be
pointed out. Several of them do not show a very impressive
drop in total mortality with moderate drinking, suggesting
death from other causes creeps up with moderate drinking.
The increase in death from other causes is striking with high
alcohol consumption.

The majority of surveys tabulated drinking habits for a
large group of volunteers and then noted mortality for the
succeeding 5 to 20 years. In four studies prior drinking
habits of the volunteers were assessed. They discovered
ex-drinkers had high CVD death rates. Nevertheless, for
statistical analysis, very few of the studies distinguished
between ex-drinkers and lifelong non-drinkers. They were all
classified as non-drinkers. This would make it appear that
not drinking somehow causes higher death rates, when in
actuality, it is the ex-drinkers that have the high death
rates.

Sharper et.al. in 1988 explored this relationship further
in the 7735 man British Regional Heart Study. They separated
lifelong non-drinkers from ex-drinkers and discovered
lifelong non-drinkers do not have higher mortality than
moderate drinkers. They found most men became ex-drinkers
because of pre-existing disease. Men who were advised,

because of illness, to quit drinking by a physician had the highest mortality. The authors summarize their results as follows: "The data suggest that the observed alcohol-mortality relationships are produced by pre-existing disease and by the movement of men with such disease into non-drinking or occasional-drinking categories. The concept of a 'protective' effect of drinking on mortaltiy, ignoring the dynamic relationship between ill-health and drinking behavior, is likely to be ill founded." An editorial in the same issue of the Lancet used stronger language in their title: "Alcohol and Mortality: The Myth of the U-Shaped Curve."

Alcohol's effect on blood lipids supports, for the most part, a protective role for alcohol. Castelli et. al. analysed data from five different studies on over 3800 subjects. They found a significant relationship between alcohol consumption and the serum levels of the protective HDL. They also found an inverse relationship with alcohol and the atherogenic LDL. Castelli's paper provides impressive evidence alcohol influences both HDL and LDL in a beneficial fashion. There was a much weaker relationship between alcohol and serum triglycerides.

Three years later, Ernst et. al. published the results of the Lipid Research Clinics Program Prevalence Study. They confirmed Castelli's work by finding a strong positive correlation between alcohol and HDL in 4855 subjects. They reported no relationship between dietary saturated fat, unsaturated fat or cholesterol and HDL levels.

There have been few controlled clinical interventions measuring the HDL response when alcohol is added to the diet. Thronton et. al. reported significant (17%) increases in HDL after 6 weeks in volunteers who consumed the equivalent of three beers daily. Camargo et.al., in a controlled alcohol study, found apolipoprotein A-1 was significantly raised or lowered by raising or lowering alcohol intake. Apolipoprotein A-1 appears to be the protective protein part of HDL, in fact it is probably a more powerful risk predictor than HDL.

Another line of evidence on platelet aggregation and fibrinolytic activity (clot dissolving ability) supports a beneficial role for alcohol. Persons consuming large amounts of alcohol have decreased platelet aggregation and increased fibrinolytic activity. Recent tissue culture work with endothelial cells demonstrated alcohol increased a substance called plasminogen activator. Plasminogen activator accelerates fibrinolytic activity.

Several autopsy studies on a total of 1800 persons have found less atherosclerosis in heavy and moderate drinkers than abstainers. Coronary arteriography studies have also reported less atherosclerosis in drinkers compared to teetolers. Animal investigations on rabbits and primates reported reduced atherosclerosis when ethanol was given along with dietary cholesterol compared to animals without ethanol.

SUMMARY and RECOMMENDATIONS: ALCOHOL

We can see a substantial body of evidence supports moderate drinking as an important protective factor. Much of the original support was epidemiological, but that is being eroded away by the finding that ex-drinkers are at much higher CVD risk. Most of work that followed the epidemiology provided a biological rational explaining why alcohol was protective.

The only really important question is 'Does alcohol save lives?' For a number of years people thought epidemiology gave a 'yes' answer. That answer is now unclear. There are no controlled prevention trials to help us here either. Without a clear answer on this question it is very difficult to recommend a patient begin moderate drinking for its health effects. Having clear evidence of benefit is especially critical for alcohol because, unlike the other possible protective factors we have looked at in this book, alcohol can do harm.

Excessive alcohol consumption causes untold misery for millions of victims and their families in addition to the enormous amount of lost income. Alcoholism sharply increases total mortality rates, cardiovascular death rates, and automobile deaths, in fact over half of all auto deaths are caused by alcohol. Alcoholics also develop a characteristic cardiomyopathy along with arrhythmias and sudden heart death.

REFERENCES

MILK

Clifford, A. et. al. Homogenized bovine milk oxidase: a critique of the hypothesis relating to plasmalogen depletion and CVD. Am J Clin Nutr 38:327-32,1983

Howard, A. and Marks, J. Hypocholesterolaemic effect of milk. Lancet 2:255,1977.

Howard, A and Marks, J Effect of milk products on serum cholesterol. Lancet 2:957,1979.

Mann, G. A factor in yogurt which lowers cholesteremia in man.   Athero 26:335-40,1977.

Ward, P et. al. Isolation of an inhibitor of hepatic cholesterolgenesis from human milk.   Athero 41:185-92,1982.

ALCOHOL

Alderman, E. and Coltart, D., Alcohol and the Heart. Br Med Bull 38:77-80,1982.

Anonymous, Alcohol and mortality: the myth of the U-shaped curve.   Lancet 2:1292-3,1988.

Camargo, C. et.al.   Effect of moderate alcohol intake on serum apolipoproteins A-I and A-II. JAMA 253:2854-7,1985

Castelli, W. et. al. Alcohol and Blood Lipids. Lancet 2:153-5,1977.

Gordon,T. et.al. Diet and Its Relation to Coronary Heart Disease and Death in Three Populations. Circ 63:500-15,1981.

Ernst, N. et. al. The Association of Plasma HDL Cholesterol with Dietary Intake and Alcohol Consumption. Circ 62(suppl IV) IV-41-52,1980.

laPorte, R. et. al. The Relationship of alcohol Consumption to Atherosclerotic Heart Disease. Prev Med 9:22-40,1980.

Laug, W. Ethyl Alcohol Enhances Plasminogen Activator Secretion by Endothelial Cells. JAMA 250:772-6,1983.

Pomrehn, P. et. al. Ischemic Heart Disease Mortality in Iowa Farmers.   JAMA 248:1073-6,1982.

St.Leger, A. et.al. Factors Associated with Cardiac Mortality in Developed Countries with Particular Reference to the consumption of Wine. Lancet 1:1017-20,1979.

Shaper, A. et.al.   Alcohol and mortality in British men: explaining the U-shaped curve. Lancet 2:1267-73,1988.

Thornton, J. et.al. Moderate Alcohol Intake Reduces Bile Cholesterol Saturation and Raises HDL Cholesterol. Lancet 2:819-21,1983.

Turner, T. et. al. The Beneficial Side of Moderate Alcohol Use.   Johns Hopkins Med J 148:53-63,1981.

11. GARLIC, CARNITINE and CSA

GARLIC

The City of Gilroy can attest to the popularity of garlic. Over 120,000 people flood this small town every year to enjoy the food and ambience of the stinking rose at its annual Garlic Festival. There is also interest in garlic and onion as a prophylactic for the cardiovascular system. In addition, reports appear in the scientific literature with increasing frequency on garlic as a natural antibiotic, in fact, a review has appeared in Medical Hypothesis on garlic as an antibiotic.

Garlic and onion are inhibitors of platelet aggregation in humans and animals. A number of trials have shown this effect on human subjects after ingestion of whole garlic, onion or their essential oils. The antiaggregating component of garlic, methyl allyl trisulphide (MATS), has been isolated and characterized. MATS has impressive anti-thrombotic and anti-aggregating activity. The anti-aggregating activity of garlic is also due in part to its ability to inhibit the production of aggregating prostaglandins. A major disadvantage with garlic and onion is the large amount used in the trials: 3 cloves of garlic (10g or 1/3rd ounce) to inhibit platelet aggregation. Animal work has supported the inhibition of platelet aggregation found in humans. Inhibition of platelet aggregation is an extremely important effect.

156 Garlic, Carnitine and CSA

Many animal experiments on rats and rabbits using garlic and onion have reported reduced serum lipids, especially when they are on high cholesterol diets. Increased HDL and reduced LDL has also been reported. The amounts of garlic or garlic extract were quite large. In one trial, rats were given 5 grams of garlic per day and in another, rabbits were administered essential oil of garlic extracted from 25 grams of whole garlic. On a weight adjusted basis for humans these would be staggering amounts (would you believe a pound of garlic or essential oil extracted from 5 pounds of garlic!). An additional important finding is garlic and onion supplementation appears to inhibit and regress experimental atherosclerosis in rabbits.

Human experiments for the most part have shown garlic or the essential oil of garlic improves blood lipids. Bordia reported the effect of 15 mg of essential oil of garlic (15 mg of essential oil is equivalent to 30 grams of whole garlic) on 20 healthy volunteers. After 6 months, serum cholesterol dropped 16%, triglycerides 20% and HDL increased 40%. He also did a controlled trial on 62 CHD patients and reported a 23% fall in serum cholesterol after 10 months on 15 mg of essential oil of garlic compared to controls. These are extremely impressive effects.

Fibrinolytic activity is greatly enhanced in animals using garlic, onion or their essential oils. Usually after a high fat meal fibrinolytic activity decreases, but if garlic or onion is added to the high fat meal, fibrinolytic activity is substantially increased. A number of trials on humans have shown this effect, with increases in fibrinolytic activity of 50 to 90%. This remarkable effect has been reported with raw, boiled (60 grams) or fried (60 grams) onions, raw or fried garlic (30 grams) or essential oil of garlic.

An interesting dietary survey of vegetarians in a Jain community in India was reported by Sainani et. al. The subjects were classified as frequent users of garlic and onion, occasional users or abstainers. They were matched for age, weight, sex and social status. The average serum cholesterol for the three groups in order of increasing garlic and onion consumption was 208, 172 and 159 mg%, the average serum triglyceride for the groups in the same order was 100, 75 and 52 mg%. The authors claim the diets and lifestyles were very similar except for garlic and onion. They conclude chronic consumption of garlic and onion has an important effect on lowering serum cholesterol and triglyceride.

Two reports by Arora et. al. do not support a very beneficial role for garlic and onion. One study used garlic or onion after a high fat meal and measured blood lipids, coagulation parameters and fibrinolytic activity 4 to 8 hours later. They found garlic produced a very moderate benefit in clotting time and fibrinolytic activity, but no benefit for blood lipids. The second study was done on 30 CHD patients and 20 healthy volunteers for 12 weeks. They reported no changes in any of the above parameters after 12 weeks of garlic therapy. It should be pointed out the dose of garlic oil was only 3.6 mg per day compared to 15 mg per day in the successful trials. Secondly, there was an extremely frequent incidence of side effects, for example, 16% of the subjects dropped out because of vomiting or diarrhea. Altogether, 60% of the subjects reported nausea, anorexia or diarrhea as side effects. This indicates there was something very unusual about the sujects in this trial or the garlic used.

The only double blinded controlled trial using garlic on humans appeared in 1987. Barrie et. al. gave 18 mg of garlic oil (extracted from 9 grams of fresh garlic) vs placebo to 20 healthy volunteers for a four week period. The results were quite remarkable. Serum cholesterol was lowered 16% compared to no significant change for placebo. HDL levels rose an amazing 23% (56 to 69 mg/100ml). Mean blood pressure was significantly lowered from 94 to 88 mmHg. There is one study on rats demonstrating lower blood pressure with garlic also. If Barrie et. al.'s results are confirmed and extended, then garlic would rank as an important front line weapon against cardiovascular disease.

SUMMARY and RECOMMENDATIONS: GARLIC

Garlic and onion inhibit platelet aggregation. An anti-aggregating substance has been isolated from garlic. Also, garlic inhibits the production of "bad" prostaglandins. In animals and humans, garlic or essential oil of garlic reduces serum cholesterol, serum triglyceride and blood pressure, while it increases fibrin dissolving activity and the beneficial lipoprotein HDL. The main problem is the amount of garlic needed to produce a theraputic effect is quite large, although garlic oil capsules seem to work as well. If one likes and uses garlic and onion there is sufficient evidence to support continued use of these flavorful herbs.

CARNITINE

Carnitine, a small molecule composed of several amino acids, is absolutely essential for the metabolism of fat. Fatty acids combine with carnitine to be transported across mitochondria membrane into the matrix of mitochondria. In the matrix, fatty acids are oxidized to release energy for muscle contraction, heat, protein synthesis and other energy requiring processes. When you consider heart and striated muscle use fat almost exclusively as an energy source, you realize the critical role carnitine plays in cardiac and skeletal muscle function. Carnitine is concentrated in and vital for the function of muscle and the metabolism of brown adipose tissue, a tissue which specializes in heat production. An interesting finding in feeding studies of laboratory animals is those animals with adequate amounts of brown adipose tissue do not become obese, but those with deficient amounts do gain excessive weight.

There is evidence for two other roles for carnitine. It is necessary for the breakdown and subsequent energy release of certain amino acids. Also, it plays an important role in the conversion of lactate into glucose by the liver, a process called gluconeogenesis. Lactate is made by muscles when glucose is burned under anaerobic conditions, a situation encountered during hypoxia and vigorous muscle use. Carnitine is made primarily by the liver and kidney, so it is not normally considered a vitamin or essential dietary substance, although deficiencies in children and adults in various disease states have been well documented. Two essential amino acids, lysine and methionine, are necessary for the sythesis of carnitine, as are iron and vitamins C, B6 and niacin. Animals put on a lysine deficient diet have reduced carnitine concentrations. Guinea pigs on low vitamin C regimens have drastically reduced carnitine levels. In fact, carnitine was substantially depressed before symptoms of vitamin C deficiency appeared in the guinea pigs. If carnitine is given orally to guinea pigs on a vitamin C deficient diet, they live longer than comparable animals without carnitine. It is possible the exhaustion and fatigue preceeding human scurvy is due to muscle carnitine deficits. Experiments have also shown carnitine depletion during niacin and vitamin B6 deficiencies.

Infants pose a special problem with carnitine nutrition. Oxidation of fat using carnitine is critical for infant survival and well being. Studies on rats and humans reveal very little carnitine is synthesized by the liver during infancy, meaning a dietary source is required. Carnitine occurs exclusively in animal protein, hence soy based milks do not contain it. Infants fed soy milks have significantly lower plasma carnitine values than those fed human or bovine milk. Human and animal milks are sources of carnitine, as is any animal protein, especially red meat. Fruits, vegetables, grains and plant products do not contain carnitine.

ANIMAL WORK: CARNITINE

Truly remarkable protective properties of carnitine have been documented in animals with ischemic myocardium. In dogs with ligated coronary arteries, there is a high incidence (9 out of 25 dogs) of ventricular fibrillation, elevation of the S-T segment of the electrocardiogram, decreased tissue levels of ATP and creatine phosphate. If dogs are infused with carnitine during the ischemic period, there is normalization of the S-T segment, no decreased levels of vital ATP or creatine phosphate and a low incidence of fibrillation (1 out of 25 dogs). The protective effect of the 5 minute carnitine infusion lasted up to 60 minutes.

During ischemia, free fatty acid concentrations increase, which causes further impariment of the heart's output. Free fatty acids directly and indirectly inhibit enzymes involved in muscle contraction. In an experiment on 45 ischemic and free fatty acid supplemented swine hearts, carnitine infusions dramatically improved mechanical heart function compared to controls without carnitine.

Another change during ischemia in rat or dog hearts is profound free and total carnitine loss if the ischemia is maintained ten minutes or longer. During the first five minutes of ischemia, often called the "reversible" phase of ischemia, no carnitine is lost. Clearly, not only does exogenous carnitine profoundly protect against myocardial deterioration during ischemia, but ischemia itself causes significant loss of this protective factor.

HUMAN WORK: CARNITINE

Human work has complimented the animal experimentation. Recently it was reported the free carnitine levels in heart muscle of patients with chronic heart failure due to mitral valve disease was strikingly lower (868 vs 382 nmole/g wet tissue) than persons without heart disease. In a controlled study of 21 coronary artery disease patients, carnitine administration significantly improved pacing endurance and heart output. A number of reports also claim L-carnitine supplementation benefits cardiomyopathic patients. For example, normal thickness of the left ventricle returned, as did normal EKG and cardiac performance after carnitine supplementation.

Eight angina patients in another study had increased work tolerance and reduction of angina with intravenous carnitine. An additional trial with 18 coronary artery disease patients confirmed IV carnitine's ability to increase exercise and work tolerance. A further study showed daily oral administration of 3.5g (50mg/kg) of carnitine significantly reduced angina attacks and nitroglycerine consumption in a 60 day controlled trial on coronary artery disease patients.

Serum lipid concentrations appear to be improved with oral carnitine. In a recent 15 week trial on two persons with low HDL levels, one gram of L-carnitine per day increased HDL by 78% and lowered triglyceride values. Pola et. al. in 1980 reported 3 grams of oral carnitine significantly reduced serum cholesterol and triglyceride in patients with type II and IV hyperlipoproteinemia. Certainly these are exciting leads which need to be confirmed in larger trials.

Even though carnitine is synthesized by kidney and liver, carnitine deficiencies do occur in malnourished and diseased persons. Animal work demonstrates carnitine status is impaired if there is inadequate intake of any of the following: lysine, methionine, vitamins B-6, C and niacin. There is no reason to suggest this impairment wouldn't occur in humans with inadequate intake of the same nutrients.

Animal protein, primarily beef and sheep muscle, has substantial amounts of carnitine, ranging from 60mg/ 100grams for lean beef muscle to 200mg/100grams of lean sheep muscle. Much smaller amounts occur in liver (2mg/100grams), chicken (1mg/100grams), milk (4mg/8oz) and eggs (0mg/100grams). Vegetable products have negligible amounts.

SUMMARY and RECOMMENDATIONS: CARNITINE

Several experiments demonstrate carnitine provides startling protection for animals hearts when faced with oxygen deprivation. Oral and intravenous experiments on humans reported carnitine decreased angina, increased heart output and work tolerance in heart disease patients. These effects are probably due to carnitine's central role in heart muscle energy metabolism. In addition, several trials report oral carnitine reduces serum cholesterol and triglyceride and raises the protective HDL.

Even though carnitine is made by the kidney and liver, supplements protect animal and human hearts. Vitamins B-6, C and niacin are required for the synthesis of carnitine. This is another reason to consume a nutrient rich diet.

CSA: A MUCOPOLYSACCHARIDE (MPS)

Mucopolysaccharides are often called glycosaminoglycans. They are an extremely complex group of compounds, widely distributed in connective tissue, forming the major portion of the 'ground substance'. They are long chain polysaccharides made of repeating sugar units, with each unit containing an amino group.

There are several different MPSs, a few of which will be briefly mentioned here. Hyaluronic acid is the most abundant member of the group and is commercially prepared from umbilical cord. Chondroitin-4-sulfate (CSA) and chondroitin-6-sulfate are found in cartilage and in the connective tissue of skin, cornea and blood vessel walls. There are also MPSs in certain plants, including red seaweed. Another MPS is heparin, well known for its anticoagulant properties.

The various mucopolysaccharides bond with proteins to form a class of molecules called proteoglycans. They are easily extracted from cartilage with an aqueous salt solution. The molecular weight of the protein part of the proteoglycan averages 16,000 and the mucopolysaccharide chain molecular weights range up to 100,000. Studies have shown between 10 and 100 mucopolysaccharide chains link to one protein, which make the proteoglycans very large and complex molecules with molecular weights in the millions.

ANIMAL STUDIES

There is good evidence to demonstrate some of the ingested mucopolysaccharides are absorbed intact from the small intestine into the blood stream. Oral administration of chondroitin-4-sulfate (CSA) to dogs and rats resulted in undegraded CSA in the blood after 30 minutes, reaching a maximum after 60 minutes and then slowly decreasing for ten hours. A feeding experiment with mice showed 40% of the CSA was absorbed in 24 hours and whole CSA was detected in the blood. Studies on isolated rabbit intestine also indicate undegraded CSA passes through the intestinal wall.

CSA has been shown to inhibit calcification of soft tissues, including arterial walls. Intravenous CSA reduces the red blood cell sedimentation rate of rats fed high fat and cholesterol diets. Heparin and other mucopolysaccharides, such as CSA, have long been known to have anticoagulant and antithrombogenic properties. CSA inhibited clot formation in rats, dogs and rabbits.

A number of workers have reported intravenous injections of CSA prevented atherosclerotic lesions of the coronary artery and aorta in rats fed special diets to induce atherosclerosis. The same prevention of vascular disease was observed in rats fed 1% CSA in their atherogenic diet. The lesions were prevented in 18 out of 18 male rats and 13 out of 18 female rats after six weeks on the diet. Vascular lesions were prevented in rabbits fed atherogenic diets by subcutaneous injections of CSA. Monkeys put on high lipid diets were protected by CSA given under the skin. The monkeys had less atherosclerosis, lower serum lipid levels and increased collateral circulation in the heart.

Morrison et. al. reported the regression of naturally occuring coronary artery disease in 8 year old monkeys given CSA subcutaneously. These authors claimed this was the first time naturally occuring (not experimentally induced) athero-sclerosis has been regressed by any agent.

HUMAN WORK

Morrison treated a total of 134 heart disease patients with oral and parenteral doses of CSA during the period 1942 to 1955. Three fourths of the patients were considerably improved, regardless of whether they were on an oral or parenteral regimen. In 1973 Morrison and Enrich published the results of a six year controlled secondary prevention trial using CSA orally. Sixty randomly selected patients with coronary heart disease were treated using conventional therapy and 60 randomly selected patients with coronary heart disease were treated with oral CSA plus conventional therapy. They were given 10 grams of the cartilage extract daily for three months, the 1.5 grams daily for four years and finally 0.75 grams for 18 months. In the CSA treated group there were 6 acute cardiac incidents including 4 deaths, but in the control group there were 42 acute cardiac incidents including 14 deaths. The reduced number of cardiac incidents and deaths in the CSA was statistically significant.

The remarkable results show an extract of cartilage given orally is highly effective in preventing coronary events in known coronary heart disease patients. The CSA was well tolerated by all patients with no side effects or complications due to medication. The CSA patients claimed they felt better, with less fatigue and improved exercise tolerance. Further, the thrombosis formation time was greatly increased for the CSA patients. In 1974 Morrison and Schjeide publish-ed a complete monograph detailing the considerable evidence supporting the use of CSA in preventing and treating cardio-vascular disease. A second monograph appeared in 1984.

In 1983 Morrison published a book titled, "Dr. Morrison's Heart Saver Program" where he discusses his ten ingredient Institute Formula (Instutute for Arteriosclerosis Research, Loma Linda University School of Medicine, Loma Linda, Ca) for preventing and treating heart disease. The tenth ingredient is mucopolysaccharide. In his work discussed above he used MPS extracted from shark or gristle which was primarily CSA. His Institute formula now uses red seaweed as their source of MPS-CSA. Morrison also includes in his book more recent results of the beneficial effect of his Institute Formula on heart disease patients. These results are unpublished and mostly uncontrolled.

SUMMARY and RECOMMENDATIONS: CSA

Animal experiments demonstrate oral or intravenous CSA is protective against atherosclerosis. It also has antithrombogenic properties and it inhibits calcification. Human clinical trials have shown remarkable protective effects.

CSA is a component of connective tissue. Americans tend to eat muscle meat and eschew gristle. These results suggest gristle should be eaten and not thrown away. Work on guinea pigs indicate vitamin C is necessary for the synthesis of CSA. This is another possible reason for the importance of vitamin C in arterial health. Dr. Morrison now uses an MPS-CSA complex which they obtain from red seaweed.

REFERENCES

GARLIC

Ariga, T. et. al. Platelet Aggregation Inhibitor in Garlic. Lancet 1:150,1981.

Arora, R. et. al. The Long-Term Use of Garlic in Ischemic Heart Disease. Athero 40:175-9,1981.

Arora, R. & Arora, S. Effect of Clofibrate, Garlic and Onion on Alimentary Hyperlipemia. Athero 39:447-52,1981.

Barrie, S. et. al. Effects of Garlic Oil on Platelets, Serum Lipids and BP in Humans. J Orthomolec Med 2:15-21,1987

Bordia, A. & Verma, S. Effect of Garlic on Regression of Atherosclerosis in Rabbits. Artery 7: 428-37,1980.

Boullin,D. Garlic as a Platelet Inhibitor. Lancet 1:776,1981

Chutani, S. & Bordia, A. Fried versus Raw Garlic on Fibrinolytic Activity in Man. Athero 38: 417-21,1981.

Kawakishi, S. & Morimitsu, New Inhibitor of Platelet Aggregation in Onion Oil.(Letter) Lancet 2:330, 1988

Lau, B. et. al. Allium Sativum (Garlic) and Atherosclerosis: A Review. Nutr Res 3:119-28,1983.

Makheja, A. et. al. Inhibition of Platelet Aggregation and TXA-2 Synthesis by Onion and Garlic. Lancet 1:781,1979.

Vatsala,T. et.al. Effects of Onion in Induced Atherosclerosis Artery 7:519-30,1980.

CARNITINE

Anonymous, Carnitine, clue or cure? Lancet 2:1027-8,1982.

Bahl, J. & Bressler, R. The Pharmacology of Carnitine. Ann Rev Pharmacol Toxicol 27:257-77,1987.

Borum, P. Carnitine. Ann Rev Nutr 3:233-59,1983.

Folts, J. et. al. Protection of the ischemic dog myocardium with carnitine. Am J Cardio 41:1209-14,1978

Liedtke, A. and Nellis, S. Effects of carnitine in ischemic swine hearts. J Clin Invest 64:440-7,1979.

Pola, P. et. al. Carnitine in the therapy of dyslipidemic patients. Curr Ther Res 27:208-15,1980

Rossi & Siliprandi. Effect of carnitine on HDL cholesterol: Report of two cases. Johns H Med J 150:51-4,1982.

Shug, A. et. al. Changes in tissue levels of carnitine during myocardial ischemia. Arch Biochm Biop 187:25-33,1978.

Suzuki, Y. et. al. Myocardial carnitine deficiency in chronic heart failure. Lancet 1:116,1982.

CHONDROITIN SULFATE A (CSA)

Morrison, L. Dr. Morrison's Heart Saver Program St. Martins Press, New York, 1983

Morrison, L. and Schjeide, O. Coronary Heart Disease and The Mucopolysaccharides. Thomas Pub. Springfield, Ill. 1974.

Morrison & Schjeide. Arteriosclerosis. Thomas Pub. Springfield, Ill. 1984

Muthiah, P. Proteoglycans and atherosclerosis: A review. Artery 4:183-202, 1978.

12. SODIUM and HYPERTENSION

We are to a topic most people assume is well established and agreed upon. I wish that were the case, because it would make the writing job much easier. Frankly, there is so much controversy on salt, I hesitate to begin. To give you a feeling for the controversy, here are some quotes from leading experts. "Sodium reduction must remain a general health goal for our nation", Hull Hayes, jr, FDA commissioner. "This whole thing has gone too far. Its a great misconception that telling Americans to reduce their sodium consumption is a public service", Dr. John Laragh, Cornell Medical School. "On the basis of current evidence, it does not appear justifiable or appropriate to undertake large-scale salt restriction in the general population to prevent hypertension.", Robert Holden et. al. JAMA 250,369,1983. "When considering sodium intake and hypertension, we still have more questions than answers", Dr. James Hunt, Ann. Int. Med. 98:724,1983. "The importance of sodium in hypertension is being dangerously minimized. I think enough is known about sodium so that we can say something ought to be done now. The sodium consumption of the population ought to be reduced", Mordecai Blaustein, U. Maryland Medical School. "Sodium restriction as a broad public health measure might actually harm more

people than it helps", Dr. David McCarron, Oregon Health
Sciences U. Now lets look at some of the issues on salt.

Sodium is an essential nutrient. Ordinary table salt,
sodium chloride, is the most common source of sodium. Fruits
vegetables, grains and natural plant products are normally
very low in sodium. Any person or culture subsisting on
plants, without added salt, would consume between 100 mg and
400 mg of sodium per day. Cultures habitually ingesting this
extremely low amount of sodium appear to be healthy and not
adversely affected by the low salt intake. Based on this and
other estimates of need, the minimum sodium requirement for
humans is thought to be 100 mg to 200 mg per day. Sweating,
fever, growth, diarrhea, vomiting, and diabetes can greatly
increase this minimum requirement.

Animal products contain considerably more sodium than plant
products. This is why the estimated average consumption of
sodium naturally occuring in all foods in a normal Western
diet is between 1000 mg (1 gram) and 2000 mg (2 grams). (It
takes 2.5 grams of table salt to provide 1 gram of sodium).
Industrial processing (making bread, canned goods, potato
chips etc.) add another 1000 to 2000 mg of sodium per day to
the diet, resulting in 2000 mg to 4000 mg of sodium consumed
per day by the average person before any salt is added at the
table or in cooking. Another 1000 mg to 2000 mg is added
during cooking or at the table, which brings the total amount
between 3000 and 7000 mg of sodium per day.

Recent evidence from England (James et.al.) shows 10% of
the sodium intake occurs naturally in food, 75% is added by
manufacturers and only 15% is discretionary use in cooking or
at the table. This indicates eliminating salt at the table
or in cooking has very little influence on salt consumption.

We can see from the above information, unless one becomes
a strict vegetarian and consumes no processed foods (breads,
canned goods, prepared meals, cakes, snacks, and candy), it
is very difficult to get below 2000 mg per day. Even to
arrive at 2000 mg per day means no added salt in cooking or
at the table and avoidance of highly salted foods such as
ham, potato chips, salted nuts and similar snacks.

These numbers help to illustrate one reason for the conflicting opinions on sodium. You see there is good evidence
diets containing 200 to 400 mg of sodium are effective in
lowering blood pressure in hypertensives. At the other

extreme, diets above 16,000 mg (16 grams) of sodium will raise blood pressure, even in normotensives, but in between these extremes, the evidence is much less consistent or convincing.

In order to get down to 400 mg, major dietary changes need to be made, ie. avoid dairy products, meats, all processed foods and salt at the table. No agency can really recommend that to 220 million people, but even if they did, who would follow it? Indeed, there are real dangers in advocating this type of severe sodium restricted diet to everybody. The most obvious problems would be protein and multiple nutrient deficiencies in a large percentage of the population. To avoid the deficiencies and properly enact a low sodium diet, a massive program of intensive, detailed nutrition education would be needed. This, of course, would be good, but the likelihood of this occuring is remote.

If severe restriction can not be promulgated, then more moderate cutbacks would seen to be in order. Most authorities advocating restrictions are suggesting a drop to 1500 to 3000mg of sodium per day from our present 3000 to 7000mg per day. Unfortunately, it is in this area of intake where there is the least evidence of benefit, hence the sharp differences of opinion on advocating sodium restriction.

Interest in sodium and hypertension dates back to 1904 when Ambard and Beaujard reported good results in severe hypertension with salt restriction. For the next 40 years a number of papers claimed moderate to excellent benefit in hypertensives on extremely low salt diets. In 1944 Kempner published the results of his celebrated rice-fruit diet. In the severe hypertensives in his trial, 60% had significant blood pressure lowering and 25% were normalized. Many researchers argued the striking benefits were due to the remarkably low (less than 230 mg sodium) sodium content of the rice-fruit diet.

The effects of other confounding factors, such as weight reduction (blood pressure lowering was greatest in obese patients), relaxation and placebo effect were not considered. Later, better controlled rice-fruit diet experiments had a beneficial response rate of 20 to 40% of the subjects instead of 60 to 70%. Trials in which there was less severe sodium restriction, in the range of 1000 mg/day, benefits of the rice fruit diet were eliminated. This was a disturbing finding, since it only takes 3 ounces of corn flakes to go from 200 mg to 1000 mg of sodium per day. Patients complained bitterly about the unpalatable fare on the rice-fruit diet and its alleged side effects of fatigue, nausea, anorexia, muscle twitching, abdominal cramps and possibly even death in some cases.

The work on sodium for the first half of this century could be summarized as follows: 1. severe sodium restriction, less than 300 mg sodium/day, is effective in lowering blood pressure in 20 to 60% of the hypertensives treated. 2. Compliance was poor because of the severity, unpalatability and side effects of the diet. 3. There was a loss of interest in moderate sodium restriction by the medical community since the 1000 mg regimens were not effective in the early trials. 4. Interest waned in the salt restricted diets because of reasons 2 and 3 and the development of effective anti hypertensive drugs. The medications were, of course, easier to administer, required no life style change and appeared to be more effective than sodium restriction.

EPIDEMIOLOGY

Dahl and Love first reported on sodium intake in various Western and non-Western countries and hypertension in 1954. They and others concluded that in cultures where sodium intake is below 700 mg, hypertension is very rare. Incidence rises to about 3% in cultures consuming between 700 mg and 1400 mg daily, which is considerably lower than our 10 to 15% hypertensive rate and 3000 to 7000 mg sodium intake. The interpopulation studies, at first sight, strongly suggest sodium intake is an important factor in hypertension, but they are not without important criticism.

The interpopulation epidemiology has been severely criticized because of: 1. the variation and unreliability of the sodium estimates. 2. the variability in definition of hypertension. 3. poor documentation of incidence. 4. confounding variables such as weight, age, activity, stress, and other dietary factors were not considered. For example, the low sodium countries, in general had high physical activity, low weight, and high calcium, magnesium and potassium intakes. 5. The whole epidemiological relationship is flawed when more countries and societies are included. I think we can conclude the international epidemiology provides some support for the sodium-hypertension thesis, but there are many important flaws in the data.

Unfortunately, to add to the confusion, the studies on sodium within one country have rarely supported the thesis. A large number of investigations at various locations, such as Framingham, Wales, New Zealand, Japan and Connecticut have failed to show a significant difference in sodium intake between normotensives and hypertensives. In one of the latest reports by Holden et. al., 5678 persons were interviewed, representing two million adults in Connecticut, revealing no difference in blood pressure between the lowest sodium group (lowest 10%) and highest sodium group (highest 10%).

The analysis of 10,372 healthy subjects in the Health and Nutrition Examination Survey (HANES I) revealed hypertensives tended to consume less sodium than normals! The HANES I results are opposite to what is expected by the sodium-hypertension hypothesis.

Smith et.al. in a Scottish study found sodium excretion did not significantly correlate with blood pressure in 7354 subjects. In sharp contrast to the sodium data, it was shown that pulse rate, age, body mass index, alcohol consumption and potassium excretion were significantly linked with blood pressure.

In 1988, results of the massive Intersalt Study of 10,000 twentyfour hour urinary sodium samples from 52 centers in 32 countries, were reported. In 48 centers there was no relationship between median blood pressure or incidence of high blood pressure and sodium excretion. There was a relationship between sodium excretion and increase in blood pressure with age. Overall the findings in this important study were very weak for sodium. Swales in his commentary evaluated the data on sodium this way, "the most striking observation seems to be that the more complex the analysis the weaker the relation."

MODERATE RESTRICTION

Moderate changes in dietary sodium have produced varying results. Unfortunately, most of the experiments have been short term with few subjects. For example, MacGregor et. al.

recent experiment with 19 moderately hypertensive patients
lasted only 8 weeks after baseline values were taken. The
subjects were on low sodium placebo, with an average total
sodium intake of 2000 mg for 4 weeks, followed by 4 weeks of
sodium supplements with an average total consumption of 3700
mg. The average blood pressure was 7mmHg lower on the 2000
mg regimen compared to the 3700 mg diet. Nevertheless,
almost half of the subjects had insignificant responses. If
the three subjects with the greatest improvement had been
non responders, then the difference between high and low
sodium would only have been 4.4 mm Hg. This emphasizes the
problem of having few subjects in an experiment that produces
a wide range of responses.

An interesting comparison can be made with Longworth's
experience with 82 hypertensive outpatients on a two week
regimen of lowered sodium. There was no significant difference for the whole group, but 14 subjects had increased blood
pressure and 14 had decreases.

A recent controlled study on hypertensive type II diabetics
found a remarkable 20 mmHg decline in systolic BP, but not
diastolic, after one month of moderate restriction. This
study indicates hypertensive type II diabetics are very
likely salt sensitive.

Variation in response to moderate and even severe sodium
manipulation is a common theme in the reports and reviews,
although there are now several short term trials which have
shown some success with moderate restriction. A general
consensus gathered from epidemiology, severe restriction,
moderate restriction, animal work and diuretic therapy is a
certain percentage of hypertensive patients, usually between
10% and 40% will respond favorably to sodium manipulation.
The responders are usually labeled salt or sodium sensitive,
which is often suggested to be a genetic trait, although
there is no direct evidence for a genetic linkage.

NORMOTENSIVES

A general consensus is normotensives do not respond to
sodium limitations with lower blood pressure. Also, they do
not appear to have increased blood pressure upon sodium
loading below 10,000 mg (10 grams). In one loading study of
normotensives, loads of 0.2grams, 2.3 grams, 6.9 grams and
13.8 grams of sodium per day did not increase blood pressure,

but 18 grams (18,000 mg) and above did. In another report, loads below 10 grams did not raise blood pressure, but 10 grams and above did. Persons with good potassium balance appeared to be protected against high sodium loads also.

DIURETICS

The fact that blood pressures are lowered in about 25-50% of the hypertensives taking diuretics supports the notion that sodium is an important determinant of blood pressure, since one of the things diuretics do is to increase the excretion rate of sodium. Clinical trials have shown diuretics are more effective in about one third of the patients if they are concurrently put on a low salt regimen and about the same number are harmed if they are put on a high salt diet. These findings are used to support the salt-hypertension theory.

ANIMAL STUDIES

Animal studies offer some support for the theory, but it is well to remember "man is not a rat" especially in a response as complex as hypertension. Strains of rats bred to be spontaneously hypertensive are for the most part insensitive to salt intake. Dahl and Love have developed lines of salt sensitive and salt insensitive rats. The salt sensitive rats become hypertensive on an 8% salt (an enormous amount of salt) diet, but the salt insensitive ones do not. These findings are used to support the idea that salt sensitivity in humans is inherited. Actually, it does not provide support, it merely suggests inherited salt sensitivity is possible in humans. A number of other animal species have also shown salt sensitivity when given massive doses of sodium. Animal experiments on the whole indicate sodium is one component of hypertension and possibly a causal factor.

SODIUM AS A CAUSE OF HYPERTENSION

The problem of whether chronic high sodium diets cause hypertension in humans has not been well addressed. The animal studies and international epidemiology suggest high dietary sodium is a causal factor, but animal experiments are not directly applicable to humans and epidemiology is never offered as evidence of a causal relationship. Epidemiology can not distinguish between causal and non-causal factors. It merely uncovers relationships which <u>may</u> be causal. Anyway, the epidemiology within one country or culture has never found a consistent relationship between sodium intake and hypertension. The other studies discussed here have shown severe and possibly moderate sodium restriction is a useful treatment for some hypertensives. These experiments do not address sodium as a cause of hypertension.

In order to test sodium as a cause of hypertension, long term controlled studies on large numbers of normotensives need to be carried out. This is easier said than done. It would be unethical to put people on high sodium regimens long term, so the experiment would have to be designed so all subjects were on a low sodium diet, with one group receiving a placebo and the other a salt tablet to bring them up to some kind of average American intake.

Think of the difficulty in deciding the the level of sodium in the low sodium diet. Epidemiology and clinical treatment trials suggest it should be very low, but at low intakes, you would have terrible compliance, since a low salt diet means more than just eliminating the salt shaker at the table and stove, a feat which seems beyond the pain threshold of many Americans. A low sodium diet means very few animal products and no commercially made snacks, cakes, breads, prepared foods, pickeled and canned goods. Regardless of the level of salt intake, previous experience with fat manipulated trials demonstrate compliance is a major problem.

Since it would be very easy to purposely or inadvertantly ingest too much sodium, it would be necessary to measure compliance independently if the trial were to be believed. Sodium intake can be measured independently by 24 hour urine sample analysis. This analysis along with the routine medical examinations, education and training of the subjects, data collection and interviews would take enormous sums of money. In 1970 when a meaningful fat manipulated trial was being planned for coronary heart disease prevention, the cost estimators arrived at the enormous figure of 500 million dollars. A decision was made at that time not to do the large fat trial because of the cost. It seems reasonable the costs for a meaningful low sodium trial would be even greater so the likelihood of it being carried out is remote. We are left with this situation: there is very little direct information on sodium as a cause of human hypertension. The issue will probably never be resolved because of the huge costs involved in order to do a decisive trial.

The only controlled, double blinded study published so far was done on 476 new born infants for 25 weeks. One half of the infants were put on low sodium regimens, the other half on normal sodium diets. The babies on low sodium diets averaged a systolic pressure 2 mm Hg lower than the normal sodium group. These results are consistent with the theory of sodium caused hypertension, but the study needs to be confirmed and lengthened to at least several years. A major problem with using infants is the great skill required to measure their blood pressure accurately. On the other hand, moderate sodium restriction would be relatively easy to implement with infants.

ALTERING THE NATIONAL SODIUM CONSUMPTION

Since moderate restriction has had occasional success, there is more interest in putting the whole nation on a low salt regimen. At most it would help the people that become hypertensive, but only 20% of the population becomes hypertensive and out of that number only one third would be salt sensitive. Therefore at most, 6% of the population would benefit from sodium restriction. This is why there is hesitation and even criticism of the idea of putting the whole nation on a low salt diet, especially when real proof showing sodium causes high blood pressure is lacking.

Many low salt advocates readily admit the lack of proof, so they base their recommendations on two ideas: 1. Low salt diets for the whole population may have benefit and if they did, the rewards would be very great. 2. It can do no harm. The second point is worth addressing.

Can a low salt diet do harm? The answer is clearly no if one is merely refering to elimination of the salt shaker at the table and in cooking. The answer is definitely yes if the restriction approaches the levels reached in the Kempner diet, due to frank sodium deficiencies in some people and multiple nutrient deficiencies in a great many people. Another problem to consider is the supply of low sodium food could not possibly meet the demand if a large percentage of Americans switched to a low sodium diet.

At intakes above 1000 mg/day, there is little danger of sodium deficiencies, but there is still considerable risk of multiple nutrient deficits, depending on food choices. If meats, dairy products, canned foods, cold cereals and bakery goods, including bread, are restricted because of sodium, it is obvious why nutrient deficiencies could develop unless intelligent food choices were made.

Another method to implement the possible benefits of a low sodium diet is to target the advise to those persons who have sodium sensitivity. The fundamental reason why some persons are sodium sensitive has not been determined. It could be there are many reasons, with individual sets of causes for different persons. A few possibilities are: 1. Inadequate calcium intake since high excretion rates of sodium cause greater excretion of calcium, exacerbating any calcium deficit. Clinical trials have shown calcium to be effective in lowering blood pressure. 2. Inadequate potassium status. Animal work and limited human studies have reported high potassium intakes protect against high sodium diets. 3. A defect in the renin-angiotensin system. Renin is released by the kidney to conserve sodium. Salt sensitive hypertensives usually have low serum renin levels compared to normotensives. Patients with high serum renin levels usually are not helped with sodium restriction or diuretics. It is not known why persons with low plasma renin are usually salt sensitive and persons with high plasma renin are not. Determining plasma renin levels could be an effective lab test to predict sodium sensitivity. Salt sensitive persons should obviously be on low sodium diets.

SUMMARY AND RECOMMENDATIONS

The evidence on sodium is very conflicting. It probably means sodium isn't the most important factor in hypertension. Severe sodium restriction does reduce blood pressure in many hypertensives, but it is difficult to implement. Moderate restriction is easier to implement and helps some hypertensives, especially type II diabetics. The question as to whether high sodium diets cause and low sodium diets prevent high blood pressure has not been answered.

Some hypertensives are salt sensitive. They should be identified and put on low sodium diets. The data at this time does not support recommending a severely restricted sodium diet for the whole nation. The evidence for moderate restriction for the whole nation is not very persuasive. Nevertheless, we do consume much more sodium than is needed and no benefits are claimed for sodium rich diets.

REFERENCES

Dodson, P. et.al. Sodium restriction and BP in hypertensive type II diabetics. Br Med J 298:227-30, 1989.

Fregly, M. Estimates of sodium and potassium intake. Ann Int Med 98:792-9,1983.

Hofman, A. et. al. A randomized trial of sodium intake and blood pressure in newborn infants. JAMA 250:370,1983.

Holden, R. et. al. Dietary salt intake and blood pressure. JAMA 250:365,1983.

Hunt, J. Sodium intake and hypertension:a cause for concern. Ann Int Med 98:724,1983.

Ingelfinger, J. Sodium and blood pressure in infancy. JAMA 250:389,1983.

Intersalt Cooperative Research Group, Intersalt: an international study of electrolyte excretion and blood pressure. Br Med J 297:319-28, 1988.

James, W. The dominance of salt in manufactured food in the sodium intake of affluent societies. Lancet 1:426-9, 1987.

Kolata, G. Value of low sodium diets questioned. Science 216: 38,1982.

Laragh, J. and Pecker, M. Dietary sodium and essential hypertension: some myths and truths. Ann Int Med 98:735-43,1983.

MacGregor, G, Dietary sodium and potassium intake and blood pressure. Lancet 1:750,1983.

MacGregor, G et. al. Double-blind randomised crossover trial of moderate sodium restriction in essential hypertension. Lancet 1:351,1982.

McCarron, D. et. al. Blood pressure and nutrient intake in the United States. Science 224:1392-1398,1984.

Pickering, G. Salt intake and essential hypertension. Cardio-vascular Reviews and Reports 1:13,1980.

Smith, W. et. al. Urinary electrolyte excretion, alcohol consumption & BP   Br Med J   297:329-30, 1988.

Swales, J. Salt saga continued. Br Med J   297:307-8, 1988.

13. POTASSIUM and HYPERTENSION

The chemical properties of sodium and potassium are almost identical. It takes special sophisticated tecniques to separate an aqueous mixture of sodium and potassium ions because their properties are so similar, especially in solution. Nevertheless, living cells can easily distinguish and separate them. It is well known cell walls actively distinguish between sodium and potassium. Attesting to this is the high concentration of potassium inside living cells with a concurrent low concentration outside cells. The situation for sodium is reverse, that is, there is very little sodium on the inside of cells and a great deal extracellularly.

Humans have about 175 grams of intracellular potassium and only 3 grams of extracellular potassium. A similar, but reverse concentration gradient exists for sodium. These remarkable concentration differences are maintained by an active sodium-potassium pump, which pumps potassium into cells and pumps sodium out of cells. If 6% of the body's stores of potassium were to suddenly leak out into the plasma and extracellular spaces, death would ensue rapidly. Muscle contractions, nerve impulse transmission and other potassium dependent processes would cease.

Both plant and animal cells concentrate potassium, but sodium is much less prevalent in the extracellular spaces of plants than animals. This means almost all unprocessed plant foods are high in potassium and low in sodium. Animal foods don't have as much potassium, especially on a per calorie basis, but they are fairly rich in sodium. Processed foods, in general, whether they are plant or animal, are lower in potassium and higher in sodium than unprocessed foods.

HISTORICAL EVIDENCE

Man has spent the majority of his long past on low sodium and high potassium diets. Food processing, reduced fruit and vegetable consuption and the easy availability of salt during the past 100 years has changed all that. Western mans' potassium intake has fallen from around 8 grams per day to 2.5 grams per day and sodium has jumped from 0.2 grams to 5 grams per day. The ratio of sodium to potassium has gone from about 1/40 to 2/1, an astounding 80 fold increase. An interesting argument, based on animal and historical human consumption patterns, can be made for lowering sodium intake and increasing potassium consumption.

The historical knowledge does tell us two things directly: first, mankind can live on higher potassium intakes, much lower sodium consumption and the sodium/potassium ratio could be 50 to 80 times lower without risk to the majority of humans. Second, sodium and potassium consumption and the sodium/potassium ratio has changed dramatically for man. There is little question of that, although the sodium potassium ratio was probably even worse 75 years ago because of salt preserved foods.

Even though the change in the sodium/potassium ratio is undisputed, it does not mean it is the cause of hypertension in modern man. For example, we do not know the prevalence of hypertension 1000 years ago. Even if there has been an increase in hypertension, there have been many other dietary, environmental and societal changes since then. It takes controlled experiments to assess the importance of the various factors involved in human hypertension. It is not possible to do controlled (or uncontrolled for that matter) experiments on human history, hence historical knowledge cannot be used to prove the case for potassium.

ANIMAL WORK.

We have already mentioned there is considerable animal work showing high intakes of sodium causes hypertension in a percentage of animals. This percentage can be changed by appropriate breeding, resulting in salt sensitive and salt insensitive strains. When potassium is given along with salt to sodium sensitive animals, the hypertensive effects of salt are attenuated. Other animal work has demonstrated potassium reduces blood pressure in spontaneously hypertensive rats, stroke prone rats and kidney impaired rats. There is a great deal of speculation as to why high potassium diets protect against both sodium dependent and sodium independent hypertension, but there is no general agreement.

One important effect is the increased excretion of sodium on high potassium regimens. This effect is poorly understood since high potassium diets stimulate the production of aldosterone, an adrenal-cortical hormone which directs the kidneys to conserve and retain sodium.

Another effect of potassium is reduced angiotensin production, a known vasocontrictive substance. The mechanism of lowering angiotensin levels is by inhibition of renin production. Renin is required in the manufacture of angiotensin. There is also evidence high potassium levels increase the sensitivity of the pressure receptors in the aortic arch. Finally, potassium has a direct vasodilatory effect on arterioles, thereby lowering blood pressure. It is important to note the hypotensive response to high potassium only occurs in hypertensive animals. The pressure in normotensive animals is insensitive to potassium rich diets.

An unusual complicating factor is that potassium depletion causes blood pressure reduction in both normal and hypertensive animals. The hypotensive action of low potassium is poorly understood since many of the physiological changes should cause increased blood pressure. For example, sodium is retained even though there is a decrease in aldosterone production. Most investigators have reported an increase in peripheral resistance due to vasoconstriction. In addition, serum renin levels are elevated. All of these changes should cause hypertension instead of hypotension.

One uniform finding which is consistent with hypotension induced by potassium depletion is a blunted response to angiotensin's pressor action. The reasons for the restraint in angiotensins action are complex and not generally agreed upon.

Salt sensitive rats (Dahl S rats) develope kidney disease when made hypertensive with added sodium chloride. In these animals the kidney tubules are dilated, kidney arterioles are thickened, plasma flow rates reduced and nephrons damaged. If potassium is supplemented concurrently with the sodium chloride, none of the above kidney pathology occurs, even in potassium supplemented animals who remained hypertensive. This shows potassium powerfully protects against kidney damage even in the presence of high blood pressure.

A strain of rats which is salt sensitive and stroke prone (SHRsp rats) when put on a high salt, low potassium diet, has an 83% mortality rate after 17 weeks. The same breed of rat given high salt and high potassium only had a 2% mortality rate during the same 17 week period. These experiments suggest potassium offers powerful protection against stroke induced mortality.

In another series of experiments, rats were matched for identical high blood pressure, yet the potassium supplemented rats had an 86% lower mortality rate. In addition, 40% of the surviving low potassium animals had spots of cerebral hemorrhage, whereas none of the potassium supplemented survivors had any evidence of cerebral hemorrhage. These studies show potassium's ability to protect against stroke death is independent of its blood pressure lowering effect. Tobian, in his important 1988 review provides additional compelling animal evidence demonstrating potassiums powerful protective properties against stroke induced death.

Normal arterial endothelial cells secrete a substance often called endothelium derived relaxing factor (EDRF), which causes arterial smooth muscle to relax. EDRF also inhibits platelet aggregation and platelet adhesion to endothelium. Hypertensive rats secrete much lower amounts of the protective EDRF, which puts the animals at greater risk for atherosclerosis, hemorrhage and clot formation. Hypertensive animals supplemented with potassium secrete normal amounts of EDRF, which is another important benefit of a generous intake of potassium.

The animal work on potassium illustrates a few lessons on hypertension, namely, hypertension is complex, that increases or decreases in blood pressure by various agents are often poorly understood and simple answers are rarely correct. Important also is the fact that agents such as potassium can protect against the ravages of hypertension even without lowering blood pressure.

EPIDEMIOLOGY

There is little direct comparison of potassium consumption in different countries. Most of the work comparing countries has been with sodium, but it is a common and well justified practice to assume sodium and potassium consumption are inversely related, that is, countries with low sodium diets are usually high in potassium and vice versa. It is known Tibet has very low potassium intake and an unusually high incidence of stroke. China, Japan and Scotland have low potassium consumption and higher stroke rate. Also, primitive cultures consuming large amounts of potassium have virtually no hypertension.

Interestingly, there is not much evidence within one population or community demonstrating a relationship between sodium and hypertension, but there is for potassium and sodium/potassium ratios. Three studies in the U.S., with 105, 662 and 574 subjects respectively, had significant inverse correlations between hypertension and potassium excretion (which is a measure of potassium intake) or positive correlations with the sodium/potassium ratio. Even though the correlations were statistically significant, they were not particularly impressive (for the Na/K ratio the correlation coefficients were .341 and .157, for potassium the inverse correlations were -.097 and -.23). Surveys in St. Lucia and South Africa have also found an inverse correlation with potassium and blood pressure. Studies in Rancho Bernardo, California, in Honolulu and in Zutphen in the Netherlands have demonstrated significant relationships between the Na/K ratio or potassium excretion and blood pressure. Also, two reports, one in Japan and one in Scotland, documented an inverse correlation between plasma potassium and high blood pressure.

Blacks in the U.S. have a much higher incidence of hypertension than whites and this has been related to significantly lower potassium excretion and higher sodium/potassium ratios for blacks in at least six surveys. In an important study in Evans County, Georgia, white men had higher (3720 mg vs 2990 mg) sodium excretion than black men, in spite of the white mens lower blood pressure. Greater sodium excretion reflects greater intake, so this study suggests sodium is a protective factor! On the other hand, potassium excretion was also higher in whites than blacks, (1964 mg vs 938 mg), providing support for potassium as a protective factor.

Analysis of nutrient intakes in 10,372 healthy persons in the Health and Nutrition Examination Survey (HANES I) revealed higher potassium consumption in normotensives compared to hypertensives. This was a statistically significant trend. The group with potassium intake below 1200 mg had twice the rate of hypertension compared to the group with intakes above 3600 mg. HANES I provides major support for potassium as a protective factor.

Khaw and Barrett-Connor found an important inverse relationship for potassium intake and stroke related deaths in Rancho Bernardo, California. The subjects were followed for 12 years, revealing much lower stroke deaths with higher potassium intake. A 400 mg per day increase of potassium (a glass of orange juice, a potato or banana) resulted in a 40% decrease in stroke death. The incidence in women eating less than 1900 mg potassium per day was almost 2 1/2 times greater than women eating more than 1900 mg per day. Indeed there were no stroke deaths in persons consuming more than 2650 mg of potassium per day.

CLINICAL TRIALS

There have been a number of controlled trials using potassium supplements on humans. Addison's human experiments on 5 subjects in 1928 was the first report on potassium and blood pressure reduction. Priddle in 1931 also reported good results with potassium. In 1986 Svetkey reduced blood pressure 7 mmHg systolic and 4 mmHg diastolic in hypertensive men using potassium. A study by Limura et. al. on hypertensives lasting 10 days and supplementing with larger amounts of potassium, reported moderate blood pressure lowering. Kaplan, in 1985, used potassium supplements to significantly lower blood pressure in thiazide diuretic patients.

A trial by Kahm and Thron gave a 2.5 gram supplement of potassium per day (about the amount found in 3 potatoes or 1 1/2 avocados) for 2 weeks and compared the blood pressure with initial and placebo values. They reported success with a diastolic reduction of 2.4 mmHg but the placebo effect was almost as great (1.4 mm Hg). The systolic was lowered a non-significant 1.1 mmHg which was less than the placebo reduction of 2.3 mmHg. Only mild benefits were seen in this experiment.

The 1984 trial by Richards et. al. investigated short term sodium restriction and potassium supplementation on 12 mild hypertensive patients. They supplemented with 8 grams of potassium for 4 weeks, but the average blood pressure did not differ from the control value. There was wide variation in individual values, for example, six of the subjects reported blood pressure elevations and six had declines. The same pattern occured on sodium restriction, namely, no average lowering, but individually there were five elevations and seven declines. These authors are cautious about recommending low sodium, high potassium diets because of the elevations in some patients with sodium restriction and potassium supplementation.

The successful randomized trial of moderate potassium supplementation on 23 hypertensives by MacGregor also illustrates some of the problems of these small studies. On average there was a 4% reduction of blood pressure, but there were six of the 23 patients who had increases in blood pressure, one a remarkable 10%. If the patients exhibiting a pressor response were removed, then on average there would have been a 6% reduction. On the other hand, there were three patients with unusually great blood pressure lowering, one with a 27% drop and two with 14% declines. If these three unusual subjects were eliminated, a non-significant 2.2% average lowering would have been reported for the trial. It appears just a few subjects in this trial makes a very large difference. This tends to give one less confidence in the conclusions of the study. Nevertheless, when all the subjects were included there was a significant 6 mm Hg decrease in systolic blood pressure. Also seeing the growing number of trials reporting significant blood pressure

reduction using potassium supplements adds major support
for potassium as an important protective factor.

SUMMARY and RECOMMENDATIONS

National and international epidemiology offers good support
for potassium as a protective factor. Animal and cellular
experiments provide substantial evidence for potassium's
beneficial role, although the reasons for the benefit are
often unclear. Of considerable importance is potassium's
unusually powerful protection against stroke induced death
in animals which is independent of its effect on blood
pressure. There is now human evidence supporting its beneficial role in stroke prevention. The numerous clinical
trials with potassium supplements to lower blood pressure
have been small and short term. There are a variety of
individual responses to potassium supplements. Some
pressures are raised, some dramatically reduced, with the
majority experiencing moderate declines.
There is a need for much larger and longer controlled
trials on normotensives and hypertensives. At present there
is not enough human work to justify a general recommendation
of potassium supplements for the general population. There
is enough evidence to recommend potassium rich diets. This
could be accomplished by diets higher in whole grains,
legumes, fresh fruits and vegetables and lower in fat and
sugar. This advise is consistent with the other dietary
recommendations made in this book.

REFERENCES

Anonymous, Potassium supplementation in essential hypertension. Nutr Rev 46:291-4,1988

Kaplan, N. et.al. Potassium supplementation in hypertensive
patients with diuretic-induced hypokalemia. N Engl J Med
213:746-9,1985

Khaw, K. & Barrett-Connor, E. Dietary Potassium & stroke
associated mortality.   N Eng J Med 316:235-40,1987.

Khaw, K and Thom, S. Randomized double blind trial of potassium on BP in normal subjects. Lancet 2:1127,1982.

Langford, H., Dietary potassium and hypertension: epidemiological data. Ann Int Med 98:770-2,1983.

Luft, F. & Weinberger, M. Potassium and blood pressure regulation. Am J Clin Nutr 45:1289-94,1987.

MacGregor, G., et. al. Moderate potassium supplementation in essential hypertension. Lancet 2:567,1982.

McCarron, D. et.al. Blood pressure and nutrient intake in the United States. Science 224:1392-8,1984.

Richards, A. et. al. BP response to moderate Na restiction & K supplemen. in mild hypertension. Lancet 1:757-61,1984.

Tobian, L. Potassium and Hypertension. Nutr Rev 46:273-83,1988

14. CALCIUM, MAGNESIUM and HYPERTENSION

HUMAN STUDIES: CALCIUM

The role of dietary calcium in hypertension and cardiovascular disease (CVD) was rarely studied or considered before 1982. This is surprising since hard water has been associated with lower incidence of CVD deaths, both in the U.S. and throughout the world, for many years. The main factor in hard water is calcium. It has been shown repeatedly that higher amounts of calcium in drinking water are strongly associated with lower CVD mortality.

To illustrate the lack of interest in calcium before 1982, the authoritative review by Masironi and Sharper in 1981 stated: "Epidemiological evidence for an association of calcium deficiency with CVD is strong, but the possibility that the association is casual is not supported by animal and lab experiments." The situation has dramatically changed since McCarron et. al. published their findings in 1982. They compared the diets of 46 persons with recently diagnosed hypertension and contrasted them with 44 normotensive controls. There were no significant differences in sodium, potassium, fat, protein, carbohydrate or caloric consumption between the two groups, but there was a significantly lower intake of calcium (668 mg/day) in the hypertensives compared to the normotensives (886 mg/day).

A short time later McCarron analysed the U.S. Department of Health, Education and Welfare's Health and Nutrition Examination Survey I (HANES I) for a relationship between dietary calcium and hypertension. Analysis of the diets of 12,411 persons from 65 locations throughout the U.S. revealed hypertensives consumed significantly less calcium (572 mg/day) than normotensives (695 mg/day). Blacks are known to have a much greater incidence of hypertension than whites. HANES I revealed blacks consumed less calcium than whites.

McCarron et.al. reanalysed the Hanes I data in 1984 reconfirming hypertensives had less dietary calcium. They also discovered hypertensives had diets lower in potassium, vitamin C and vitamin A. Hypertensives consumed fewer dairy products and tended to consume less sodium. The values for sodium are very surprising and go against conventional wisdom.

There are other reports suggesting dietary calcium has a protective effect. Belizan and Villar reported countries with calcium rich diets had much lower incidence of eclampsia, the hypertensive crisis of pregnancy. This relationship cut across socioeconomic levels. Very poor countries like Ethiopia and Guatemala have high calcium consumption and very low eclampsia rates. In another study, Ackley et. al. showed less dairy calcium in hypertensive men compared to normotensive controls. In a controlled supplemental trial of 1 gram of calcium per day, Belizan et. al. reported a 5.6% and 9% reduction of diastolic pressure in women and men respectively. Another line of evidence comes from studies on osteoporotic women. They have a much higher incidence of hypertension than non osteoporotic controls. It is generally agreed osteoporosis is, in part, a reflection of inadequate calcium intake.

A number of controlled supplemental trials have appeared since 1984. McCarron and Morris in 1985 enrolled 48 moderate hypertensives and 32 normals in a double blind placebo controlled trial supplementing with 1000 mg of calcium for 8 weeks. They found a significant average lowering of systolic (5.6 mmHg) and diastolic (2.3 mmHg) pressure in the hypertensive group but not in the normals. Fortyfour percent of the hypertensives had systolic reductions of 10 mmHg or greater. It is important to note that pressure reductions didn't take place until after the sixth week of supplementation.

In a double blind trial, Grobbee and Hofman gave 90 mildly hypertensive subjects 1000 mg of calcium or placebo for 12 weeks. Systolic pressure was not significantly effected but after 6 weeks diastolic pressure had dropped 3 mmHg. In this study those subjects with high serum parathyroid hormone, excess weight or low serum calcium had the best response to supplements.

A four year supplemental trial of 81 normotensive and 34 medicated hypertensives was published by Johnson et. al. in 1985. There were no differences noted in the normal women, but in supplemented hypertensive women there was a 13 mmHg lowering of systolic pressure and a 7 mmHg elevation in the unsupplemented hypertensive women after 4 years. This well monitored study strongly supports a role for long term calcium supplementation in hypertensives.

There have been 3 other intervention studies which have shown a benefit with calcium. There are 4 published papers not reporting a benefit with calcium. All 4 negative reports had small sample sizes and were short term.

ANIMAL STUDIES

Moderate calcium restriction in two species of rat, one of which is bred to be spontaneously hypertensive, results in increased arterial pressure in both species and even greater calcium restriction produces hypertension. Spontaneously hypertensive rats, when given calcium supplements either during adolescence or adulthood, reduces blood pressure to near normal. Other studies have found pregnant, calcium restricted rats become hypertensive and calcium supplements reverse the condition.

Some facts on the blood pressure reducing effects of certain diuretics and sodium restricted diets fit nicely with the calcium-hypertension hypothesis. For example, the effective thiazide diuretics inhibit calcium excretion, producing positive calcium balances in patients. This has been proposed as an important, but overlooked, mechanism of thiazide's hypotensive action.

On sodium restricted diets, both sodium and calcium excretion is reduced, meaning low sodium diets improve calcium status. This could be one of the main reasons low sodium diets improves hypertension in some patients. As expected, excessive sodium caused elevated excretion rates for both sodium and calcium, meaning high sodium diets impair calcium status. A major unrecognized and possibly critical problem with salty diets is poor calcium status. The sodium-calcium relationship seems to be a two way street, because increased calcium excretion causes higher sodium excretion. On this basis one would predict calcium rich diets would protect against excessive sodium. It turns out the prediction is correct, extra calcium does protect animals against high sodium diets. There is also epidemiological evidence demonstrating calcium protects against the hypertensive effect of excess sodium.

CELL STUDIES

On the cellular level some of the actions of calcium appear at first glance to contradict calcium's hypotensive effect. For example, in order to initiate cardiac or smooth muscle contraction, calcium needs to flow into the muscle cell. The calcium combines with a substance called calmodulin, which then sets off a series of events resulting in a muscle contraction. Increased contraction of arterial smooth muscle causes higher peripheral resistance to blood flow, which is a major factor in high blood pressure. Greater contraction of cardiac muscle will produce higher heart output, which is another major factor in hypertension. One strategy to lower peripheral resistance and cardiac output is to block calciums entry into smooth muscle and heart muscle. This is the basis for the calcium antagonist drugs, which have been so successful in reducing hypertension, coronary artery spasm and cardiac contractility.

The effectiveness of the calcium antagonists would seem to argue in favor of reducing dietary calcium. If a high flow of calcium into the cell is one of the causes of hypertension, then it would appear logical to predict high calcium intakes would increase blood pressure and lower intakes would reduce blood pressure. As we have seen from dietary epidemiology and clinical trials, exactly the opposite is true.

Tissue and cellular experiments support the epidemiology. For example, in vascular tissue preparations, increased extracellular calcium concentration relaxes vascular smooth muscle cells. Furthermore, experiments have demonstrated that calcium acts as a specific inhibitor of calcium entry channels. In other words, extracellular calcium (which would correspond to blood or plasma calcium) acts as a calcium antagonist. This is a very surprising finding, but it is consistent with, indeed, supports very strongly the dietary epidemiology, clinical trials and animal work demonstrating increased dietary calcium reduces blood pressure.

SUMMARY and RECOMMENDATIONS: CALCIUM

There is now substantial epidemiology supporting dietary calcium as a protective factor against hypertension. Dairy products, being calcium rich, appear to be protective. Limited clinical trials report blood pressure reduction with calcium supplements. Animal experiments confirm calcium's protective role. On the cellular level, calcium acts as a calcium antagonist. Synthetic calcium antagonists have been successful hypotensive agents. A sensible recommendation based on the calcium evidence would be to ingest at least 800 mg of calcium a day.

The calcium RDA for adults is 800 mg. Our protein, phosphate (from soft drinks) and salt rich diets makes our calcium requirements higher than in many underdeveloped countries. Dairy products are the best sources of calcium. One cup of milk has 300 mg, one cup of plain yogurt (add your own fruit and a touch of jam if you like) contains 400 mg, and one ounce chedar cheese (remember it's 70% fat) has 200 mg. Of course, non-fat or low fat dairy products fit best with the other recommendations made in this book.

Most fruits, except oranges, are very moderate sources, usually providing less than 25 mg per serving. Green leafy vegetables and broccoli are excellent, containing between 150 and 400 mg per cup. Other vegetables and legumes range between 25 and 75 mg per serving. If supplementation is being considered, it seems 800 mg should be the maximum except with osteoporosis. Calcium carbonate, gluconate or lactate are fine. Oyster shell calcium, bone meal and dolomite should be avoided because one laboratory reported trace amounts of lead in some samples. Calcium citrate may provide better absorption, but this is a disputed finding.

MAGNESIUM

This section will deal primarily with magnesium and hypertension. There is an extensive literature on magnesium and CVD covered in Chapter 3.

World and nationwide hard water data, along with many autopsy studies reporting significantly lower heart muscle magnesium in persons dying from ischemic heart disease, have long supported the role of magnesium as a protective factor in CVD. Magnesium sulfate has been used for many years to treat the hypertensive crisis of eclampsia. McCarron reported magnesium poor diets in hypertensives (206 mg) compared to normotensives (261 mg) in a survey of 90 persons. Joffres et. al. assessed 61 dietary variables in 615 healthy men living in Hawaii. They found magnesium more associated with blood pressure than any other nutrient. Lower magnesium intake was linked with higher blood pressure.

There are three reports on human hypertensives given supplemental magnesium. Mroczeh investigated the short term effects of intravenous magnesium sulfate on cardiovascular hemodynamics in both normals and hypertensives. Peripheral resistance was reduced a remarkable 35% in hypertensives and 20% in normals. Reduction in peripheral resistance is due to relaxation of arterioles and if no other factors change, it will result in decreased blood pressure. Heart output increased in both groups about 33%. The increase in heart output was likely the reason the blood pressure did not decrease in the normotensives, but it did fall 11% in the hypertensives.

In 1985 Cappuccio reported on a two month, double blind crossover study on 17 mild hypertensives using 360 mg of magnesium. Eight had BP decreases but 9 had no change or BP increases. There was no significant benefit for the group.

Dychner and Wester gave 365 mg of magnesium to twenty hypertensives and/or congestive heart failure patients taking diuretics, comparing them with matched controls not given magnesium. The magnesium group had a significant drop in systolic blood pressure (152 mmHg to 140 mm Hg) after six months compared to no change in the controls. Note, Cappuccio above only supplemented one month.

Related to the magnesium-hypertension problem are the effects of thiazide diuretics. It is now well documented most diuretics cause greater excretion of magnesium and potential magnesium depletion. Several researchers have reported patients on diuretic therapy who are magnesium and potassium depleted with low serum sodium. These patients did not respond to oral potassium repletion therapy.

It is thought the magnesium deficiency causes the cellular potassium and serum sodium depletion since magnesium is needed for the sodium and potassium pumps. Without effective sodium and potassium pumps, potassium can not be transported into the cells and sodium can not be pumped out of the cells into the serum. In these patients, sodium and potassium supplements do not restore status unless magnesium is given along with the sodium or potassium therapy.

The potassium depletion is a dangerous situation due to the increased contractility of heart and smooth muscle. The enhanced contractility of the heart can lead to higher blood pressure, arrhythmia or fibrillation. The heightened smooth muscle contractility produces greater peripheral resistance which results in hypertension. Whang et. al. claims 50% of the potassium depleted patients are hypomagnesemic. He recommends they be supplemented with potassium and magnesium in a 8 to 1 molar ratio.

Low serum sodium caused by diuretics is not an uncommon condition. Often the condition becomes resistant to diuretic therapy. Sodium infusions exacerbate the situation by increasing thirst, edema and can lead to death. In a study using IV magnesium sulfate without sodium or potassium, the muscle potassium, serum potassium and serum sodium were raised along with a lowered muscle sodium. All of these parameters were put in normal ranges with intravenous magnesium sulfate.

Another documented effect of magnesium deficiency in humans and most animals (except the rat) is depressed serum calcium levels. The hypocalcemia produced by magnesium deficiency is not responsive to calcium supplements, but does return to normal when magnesium is provided orally. Possibly one of the benefits of adequate magnesium, in terms of hypertension, is restoration of serum calcium levels, since normal serum calcium favors normal blood pressure.

MAGNESIUM and MUSCLE CONTRACTIONS

Both animal and human work support a role for magnesium in reducing muscle contractility. For example, convulsions in animals and probably in humans are produced by magnesium deficiencies. Alcoholic and eclampsic convulsions in humans are effectively treated with magnesium sulfate. These convulsions are symptomatic of the increased irritability of hypomagnesmic muscle. It has been known for many years that magnesium deficient heart muscle in animals and humans is highly susceptible to life threatening arrhythmia and fibrillation. Many papers attest to the effectiveness of magnesium infusions to treat arrhythmia and fibrillation in animals and humans. (see Chapter 3)

The effect of magnesium on arterial smooth muscle is equally dramatic. Isolated blood vessels from many mammalian species, when magnesium deficient, produce "rapid, potent contractile responses." The opposite is true for hypermagnesmia. Arteries lose their tone with excess magnesium because of the lack of smooth muscle contraction. Many circulating neurohormones, such as catecholamines, angiotensins, acetylcholine, serotonin and vasoactive peptides have greatly increased constrictor action on magnesium deficient arteries and veins. When the magnesium concentration is raised, the contractile responses of the vessels to these circulating neurohormones are blunted.

Work on prostaglandins and beta adrenergic amines (eg isoproterenol) helps explain the increased contractility during magnesium depletion. Some of these compounds inhibit smooth muscle contraction, thereby causing blood vessels to dilate. Recent work indicates these beneficial compounds require magnesium to produce their dilating effects.

Magnesium status has a profound effect on the spontaneous tone of arteries. When the magnesium content of the fluid bathing arteries is raised, there is relaxation of muscle tone. In the same arteries, spasms are produced with magnesium deficits.

It is important to note not all arteries have spontaneous tone. Altura compared the response of various types of arteries to high and low magnesium concentration. The arteries which exhibit spontaneous tone (cerebral and coronary arteries, rat mesenteric arterioles, human umbilical vessels) respond as stated above to magnesium changes, but vessels without spontaneous tone (intrapulmonary arteries and veins, renal arteries and veins, hepatic arteries) are not affected by magnesium concentration changes.

There are several mechanisms which help explain magnesium's effect on muscle contraction. One possibility is magnesium deficiency induces decreases in cellular potassium and increases in cellular sodium. Both of these conditions produce muscle hyperirritability. Another possibility is magnesiums well documented action as a calcium antagonist. Many lines of evidence supports magnesiums role in controlling calciums influx into muscle cells. Recent work with the isotope calcium-45, provides convincing evidence for this effect. The control of calcium influx is one of the most important factors in the control of muscle contraction.

SUMMARY and RECOMMENDATIONS: MAGNESIUM

There are surveys showing people who consume less magnesium have higher blood pressure. A few clinical trials report reduced blood pressure when magnesium is administered orally or intravenously. The experiments on magnesium demonstrating arteries relax with magnesium and contract without magnesium provides a persuasive reason why magnesium should lower peripheral resistance and thereby lower blood pressure. Large clinical trials are needed to adequately test the effectiveness of magnesium as a hypotensive agent.

A typical American diet rich in fat, sugar and polished grains is usually low in magnesium. Vegetables, especially green leafy ones, whole grains, legumes and some fruits are good sources of magnesium. The other chapter on magnesium has information on RDA's, dietary sources and supplements.

REFERENCES

CALCIUM

Ackley, S. et. al. Dairy Products, Calcium and blood pressure. Am J Clin Nutr 38:457-61,1983.

Belizan, J. et. al. Reduction of blood pressure with calcium supplementation in young adults. JAMA 249:1161,1983.

Grobbee, D & Hofman, A. Effect of calcium supplementation on diastolic blood pressure. Lancet 2:703-6,1986.

Johnson, N. et.al. Effects on BP of calcium supplementation of women. Am J Clin Nutr 42:12-17,1985.

Lyle, R. et. al. BP and metabolic effects of calcium supplementation. JAMA 257:1772-6,1987.

Masironi, R. & Sharper, A. Epidemiological studies of health effects of water. Ann Rev Nutr 1:375-400,1981.

McCarron, D. Calcium and magnesium nutrition in human hypertension. Ann Int Med 98:800-5,1983.

McCarron, D. et. al. Blood pressure and nutrient intake in the United States. Science 224:1392-8,1984.

McCarron, D. & Morris, C. Blood pressure response to oral calcium. Ann Int Med 103:825-31,1985

McCarron, D. & Morris, C. The calcium deficiency hypothesis of hypertension. Ann Int Med 107:919-22,1987.

MAGNESIUM

Altura, B. et. al. Hypomagnesemia and vasoconstriction. Artery 9:212-31,1981.

Cappuccio, F. et. al. Lack of effect of oral Magnesium on high BP. Br Med J 291:235-8,1985

Dyckner, T and Wester, P. Effects of Magnesium infusions in diuretic induced hyponatraemia. Lancet 1:585-6,1981.

Dyckner, T and Wester, P. Effect of magnesium on blood pressure. Br Med J 286:1847-9,1983.

Haddy & Seelig, Magnesium & arteries in: Magnesium in Health & Disease, Cantin and Seelig, eds. Spectrum 1980, pp 639-657.

Joffres, M. et. al. Magnesium intake and blood pressure, Honolulu Heart Study Am J Clin Nutr 45:468-75,1987.

McCarron, D. Calcium and magnesium nutrition in human hypertension. Ann Int Med 98(part 2):800-5,1983.

Mroczek, W. et. al. Effect of magnesium sulfate on cardio-vascular hemodynamics. Angiology 28:720-4,1977.

Prasad, D. et. al. Magnesium deficiency produces spasms of coronary arteries. Science 208:198-200,1980.

Whang, R. et. al. Magnesium depletion as a cause of refractory potassium repletion. J Am Col Nutr 2:278, 1983.

15. WEIGHT, FIBER, LIPID, PROTEIN and HYPERTENSION

WEIGHT

It is common knowledge that obesity and hypertension are related. This has been reported in scientific studies since the 1920's. Significant correlations between weight and blood pressure are found in infancy and the correlation increases with age, reaching a maximun in the late teens and then gradually decreases with age. Both industrialized and unindustrialized societies report similar relationships between weight and hypertension in children, but in groups over 70 years old there is little systematic correlation between body weight and blood pressure.

Studies on weight-blood pressure changes in individuals suggest there is a cause-effect relationship between weight and blood pressure. Persons who gain weight, especially in young adulthood, have a high probability of subsequent hypertension and conversely, those who lose weight generally report reduced blood pressure. An unusual feature of this cause-effect relationship is it occurs with normotensives, that is, if a normotensive loses weight, in general his blood pressure goes down. This decrease does not occur in normotensives when they are given antihypertensive drugs or salt restricted diets. Antihypertensive drugs and salt restricted diets only work on hypertensives.

Stressing the importance of the weight-blood pressure relationship, Tyroler suggested, based on extensive epidemiology, that elimination of obesity would reduce the incidence of hypertension by 48% in whites and 28% in blacks. Surveys have shown weight has a closer relationship with hypertension than sodium intake. The connection between weight and blood pressure is well established. Nevertheless, the reasons for or the mechanisms behind this relationship are poorly understood and at this time there is no general consensus as to why the relationship exists.

A recent 5 month placebo controlled trial (MacMahon) on 56 overweight hypertensives showed weight loss produced greater blood pressure reduction (13 mmHg systolic, 10 mmHg diastolic) than an commonly used beta blocker anti-hypertensive drug. The weight loss had other benefits whereas the anti-hypertensive drugs usually have harmful side effects.

A four year trial (Stamler) using salt, weight and alcohol reduction resulted in normal blood pressure in 40% of the patients. Further, the final report of the Subcommittee on Nonpharmacological Therapy of High Blood Pressure listed weight reduction as a proven method for blood pressure reduction. There is also massive recent epidemiological evidence on weight and blood pressure: the 9500 person HANES survey (Gruchow), the 10,000 member Intersalt study, and the 7350 person Scottish Heart Health study (Smith).

For overweight persons with hypertension, it seems the first order of business should be to lose weight. Weight loss in overweight normotensives would be an important step to help prevent future hypertension. Permanent weight loss usually requires exercise plus moderate calorie reduction. Eliminating excessive dietary fat is the easiest way to reduce calories.

FIBER

There are several trials on humans claiming high fiber diets result in lower blood pressures. Wright et. al.'s study of 94 healthy volunteers reported lower blood pressure in people habitually consuming fiber rich diets and blood pressure reduction when fiber poor diets are changed to fiber dense diets. Further, blood pressures were raised when persons normally consuming high fiber diets were put on low fiber regimens. These trials lasted ten weeks and the maximum average blood pressure change in any group was 6.8%.

Anderson in 1982 reported a 10% average blood pressure decline in 12 diabetics (6 were normotensive, 6 were hypertensive) after they were put on a high fiber, high carbohydrate, low fat diet. Rouse et. al. also reported lower blood pressure when normotensive subjects switched to a fiber rich vegetarian diet for 6 weeks.

Unfortunately, these experiments changed many variables in addition to fiber. Rouse recently examined their high fiber, vegetarian diet and found, in addition to a 70% fiber increase, a 75% increase in polyunsaturated fats, a 20% increase in potassium, and increases of 25% for calcium, 30% for magnesium, 75% for vitamin C and 80% for vitamin E. With this many variables changing, it is difficult to conclude that fiber was the major hypotensive factor. The same problem of interpretation occurs, due to the many uncontrolled variables, when lower pressure vegetarian cultures are compared with hypertensive western cultures.

Fruits, vegetables, whole grains, legumes, and seeds are the important sources of fiber. If you consume a diet rich in fiber, there isn't much room left for sugar, polished grains, meats, or fat. As Rouse pointed out, a fiber dense diet will be nutrient dense. It may be the combination of nutrients is more important than the fiber. Nevertheless, fiber rich, vegetarian slanted diets, regardless of the reason, appear to lower blood pressure. The best way to attempt to lower blood pressure via fiber is to mimic the experiments, that is, eat high fiber foods such as fruits, vegetables, legumes and whole grains, rather than merely adding bran to a standard low fiber, low nutrient and sugar, fat and meat rich diet. A fiber rich diet combined with weight loss would be a good general strategy for blood pressure reduction.

LIPID

Two recent authoritative reviews (Goodnight and Grundy) on lipids and cardiovascular disease published in American Heart Association journals did not mention the effects of dietary lipids on blood pressure. It is very surprising that a lipid-blood pressure relationship was not discovered in any of the lipid prevention trials or the many prospective and retrospective epidemiological surveys done for the past 30 years.

There have been a vast number of lipid trials, surveys, studies, and experiments done on humans but very few, certainly none of the major ones, reported a relationship between dietary lipid and blood pressure before 1982. The lack of significant findings prior to 1982 weakens the case for the effects different fats may have on blood pressure and suggests the recent positive results with lipids should be evaluated cautiously.

The most impressive lipid-blood pressure experiment was done in Finland by Puska et. al. on 114 subjects aged 30 to 50 years, half of whom had mild untreated hypertension. They were divided into three groups: Group 1 had a high salt, low (23%) fat diet with a polyunsaturated fat to saturated fat ratio of 1/1. Group 2 was a low salt but ordinary high (43%) fat diet. Group 3 was a control with a 43% fat and high salt diet. For two weeks blood pressure measurements were made but no dietary changes were put into effect. After the two week baseline period the dietary changes commenced for six weeks after which they switched back to their pre-experimental diet for six weeks.

Groups 2 and 3 had no significant blood pressure change by the end of the six week experimental period, but Group 1 (low fat) did have a significant 8% fall in blood pressure. Their blood pressure returned to pretreatment values after switching back to their ordinary diet.

The diet apparently was effective, but the reason for its effectiveness is open to some debate. Was it the low fat per se or the low amounts of saturated fat? Further, fiber, calcium, potassium and magnesium intakes were not assessed. A possibly important aspect not addressed was the 20% reduction in calories during the experimental period for Group 1 but not for the other groups. Even with these doubts in mind, it is possible the low fat was an important variable. The Finnish researchers did a previous smaller study with almost identical results.

A number of other reports have supported the Finnish experiments. In a 40 day intervention trial with 21 people,

Iacono reported a significant decrease in blood pressure on a low fat regimen (25% fat) with a high polyunsaturated to saturated fat ratio (1/1). The low blood pressures continued when switched to a 35% fat diet with the same polyunsaturated to saturated fat ratio. In a second study, ten hypertensives and ten normotensives were put on a 25% fat diet with a polyunsaturated to saturated fat ratio of 1/1. There was a significant decrease in blood pressure in the hypertensives. Their blood pressures went back up on a high saturated fat diet. A third study with 28 males revealed a significant lowering of blood pressure on a high ratio of polyunsaturated to saturated fat regardless of whether they were low (25%) or high (43%) fat diets, although the low fat diets had the greatest response.

These experiments taken together suggest a diet with a high ratio of polyunsaturated to saturated fat, especially when it is low in total fat reduces blood pressure. A major flaw has been the lack of control over total caloric intake during the experimental verses the control periods. None of these experiments have addressed the question of long term blood pressure lowering. It is hoped a scaled up long term study will be done. If they are sucessful, we will probably have another general euphoria about lipids being the key to all aspects of cardiovascular disease. I think we can see from the information presented in this book that lipids are important, but so are many other substances.

Theoretically fish oils should lower blood pressure since they contain EPA (eicosapentanoic acid) which is a starting material for the beneficial, artery dilating prostaglandin PGI-3, but is not a starting material for harmful, artery constricting prostaglandins. Two small human experiments support a role in blood pressure reduction for fish oils. One gave cod liver oil to eight subjects resulting in reduced blood pressure.(caution: chronic high intakes of cod liver oil can produce vitamin A and D toxicity. Excessive vitamin D in animals accelerates atherosclerosis). Another experiment fed a little over one half pound of mackerel or herring to 15 normotensive subjects. The people receiving mackerel, which contains a great deal of EPA, had significant blood pressure decreases, whereas those eating herring, which does not contain as much, did not have decreased blood pressure. Salmon and mackerel have the highest amounts of EPA. One half pound of salmon contains about 30 grams of oil, 4 grams of which is EPA. Fish oils containing EPA have other beneficial effects such as lower serum triglyceride levels and decreased clotting tendency.

The limited animal experiments concerning dietary fat and blood pressure are confusing and contradictory in their results. One study reported animals on low salt diets given large amounts of polyunsaturated fats had lower blood pressure than diets with small amounts of polyunsaturated fat. Many other animal studies have shown low fat combined with low salt are more effective than adding polyunsaturated fats. In spontaneously hypertensive rats, diets with excessive saturated fat produced lower blood pressure, a very unexpected result. In other experiments using excessive salt, it appeared low fat regimens increased blood pressure, whereas high fat diets lowered blood pressure. Also on high fat diets, the effects of salt are minimized.

SUMMARY and RECOMMENDATIONS: LIPID

The results on animals are very confusing and more work needs to be done to clarify the situation. I do not think conclusions on fat and hypertension can be drawn from the animal esperiments. The human work is recent and suggests low fat diets having a high polyunsaturated to saturated fat ratio will moderately reduce blood pressure. It is puzzling why this effect was not noticed before 1982, since there have been thousands of fat trials on humans. I think if the effect of fat on blood pressure were really important, it would have been noticed many years ago. The trials on fish oils have been too small and too few to definitely conclude they lower blood pressure.

The limited experiments on humans suggest a blood pressure reduction will result from a low fat diet that has a polyunsaturated to saturated fat ratio of 1:1. This advise is the same as the recommendations based on other food factors discussed in this book. A low fat diet will be richer in vegetables, fruits, fiber, whole grains, legumes and protective nutrients.

PROTEIN

There is little evidence supporting a role for dietary protein in hypertension. International population surveys don't show a systematic relationship between protein intake and hypertension. Vegetarians in Western countries do not have significantly lower blood pressure than weight-matched controls. Feeding vegetarians meat does not significantly increase their blood pressure. Also, hypertensive animals show no effect when put on a lower protein diet.

It is important to note that chronically malnourished people are often hypotensive because of decreased cardiac output. Replenishing protein in malnourished patients usually normalizes their blood pressure, but the effect of blood pressure elevation with protein has never been found in well nourished subjects. Another important effect to keep in mind is caloric restriction and weight loss ordinarily produces blood pressure reduction, hence persons put on a low protein, calorie restricted diet will have reduced blood pressure but the effect is not due to the low protein intake.

Closely associated with blood pressure is renal function. Protein intake profoundly affects renal function. Animal and human work has convincingly demonstrated high protein diets can increase renal blood flow and glomerular filtration rates by 40 to 100%. For example, dogs fed meat meals will have dramatic kidney flow rate increases within one hour of eating and the effect persists for several hours. When the dogs are fed fat or carbohydrate meals, there is no increase in flow rates.

After eating six ounces of meat, humans have an average 50% increase in glomerular filtration rate. A study of vegetarians reported their flow rates to be one half the value of non-vegetarians. It is speculated certain amino acids stimulate the release of an unknown hormone which increases kidney flow rates.

In animals, high protein diets increase age associated glomerular sclerosis and reduced protein decreases the incidence of these lesions. In humans with normal kidney function, age associated glomerular sclerosis is not a common problem even in the eighth decade. However, studies on animals and humans with kidney disease or surgical removal of one kidney have poorer prognosis with high filtration rates. Protein reduction in these situations appears to have beneficial effects on renal function.

We can see there is little relating protein consumption directly with hypertension. Indirectly protein may affect blood pressure by increasing kidney filtration rates and possibly kidney disease. Kidney disease is a common cause of hypertension.

Advise based on the protein work would be to avoid excessive protein consumption. This is consistent with other recommendations in this book. The protein RDA for females is 46g and for males is 56g. Surveys show many adults consume more than 90 grams per day. Six ounces of lean beef or other animal flesh provides about 45 g of protein.

REFERENCES

WEIGHT

Dustan,H. Mechanisms of hypertension associated with obesity. Ann Int Med 98:860,1983.

Gruchow, H. et al. Alcohol, nutrient intake and hypertension in US adults.   JAMA 253:1567-70,1985.

Havlik, R. et. al. Weight and hypertension. Ann Int Med 98:855,1983.

Intersalt Cooperative Research Group. Intersalt. Br Med J 297:319-28,1988.

MacMahon, S. et. al. Comparison of weight reduction with Metoprolol in BP treatment.   Lancet 1:1233-6,1985.

Smith, W. et. al. Scottish heart health study. Br Med J 297:329-30,1988.

Stamler, R. et. al. Nutritional therapy for high blood pressure. JAMA 257:1484-91,1987.

Subcommittee on Nonpharmacological Therapy. Nonpharmacological approaches to BP. Hypertension 8:444-67, 1986.

FIBER

Anderson, J. Plant fiber and blood pressure. Ann Int Med 98:842-6,1983.

Rouse, I. et. al. Vegetarian diet and blood pressure. Lancet 2:742,1983.

Rouse, I. et. al. Blood pressure lowering effect of a vegetarian diet controlled trial in normotensive subjects. Lancet 1:5,1983.

Schlamowitz, P. et. al. Treatment of mild to moderate hypertension with dietary fibre. (Letter) Lancet 2:   1987.

Wright, A. et. al. Dietary fibre and blood pressure. Br Med J 2:1541,1979.

LIPID

Goodnight, S. Polyunsaturated fatty acids, hyperlipidemia and thrombosis. Arterio 2: 87-113,1982.

Grundy, S. et. al. Rationale of the diet-heart statement of the American Heart Assn. Circ 65:839A-853A,1982

Iacano, J. et. al. Reduction of BP associated with polyunsaturated fat. Hypertension 4(supp III:34,1982)

Lorenz, R. et. al. Platelet function, TXA-2 and BP with cod liver oil. Circ 67:504,1983.

Podell, R. Polyunsaturated fats and blood pressure control. Post Grad Med 74:327,1983

Puska, P. et. al. Controlled, randomized trial of the effect of dietary fat on BP. Lancet 1:1,1983.

Singer, P. et. al. Lipid and BP lowering effect of a mackerel diet in man. Athero 49:99,1983.

PROTEIN

Meyer, T. et. al. Dietary protein intake and progressive glomerular sclerosis. Ann Int Med 98:832,1983

16. CAFFEINE, ALCOHOL, SUGAR
    and HYPERTENSION

CAFFEINE

The role of caffeine in most chronic diseases is unclear and contradictory. For example, a few prospective studies report six or more cups of coffee per day doubles the risk for myocardial infarct, but in opposition to this are six studies reporting coffee is not a risk factor. The reports which show coffee to be a risk factor have been strongly criticized for poor selection of patients and controls.

There are equally contradictory findings on hypertension and caffeine. Of four early reports on caffeine and hypertension, two claimed caffeine raised blood pressure, one showed no effect and one showed blood pressure was lowered with caffeine. A similar divergence was reported for pulse rate.

A major reason for the contradictory results on blood pressure and pulse rate is the difference in response between chronic consumers of caffeine and non-consumers. For instance, a recent study showed caffeine naive subjects, when given one dose of caffeine, have elevations in blood pressure and pulse rate for a few hours. In contrast, a 7 day supplemental trial, which would mimic caffeine habituation, reported elevations in blood pressure and pulse rate the first one to four days, but after that, complete tolerance developed with no responses to caffeine noted in the subjects.

An investigation of 16 habitual smoking and coffee consuming hypertensives reported significantly lower blood pressure and pulse rate when they abstained from caffeine and cigarettes overnight. Drinking coffee in the morning slightly elevated both responses when measured one to two hours later. The combination of coffee and cigarettes produced significantly higher blood pressure after one to two hours compared to placebo. Hence the combination of coffee and cigarettes may increase blood pressure short term, but epidemiology does not support the combination of coffee and cigarettes as causing hypertension.

Ammon et. al. reported a short term increase in blood pressure in a double blind study of 10 volunteers. After several days blood pressure fell back to baseline and remained there for 4 weeks of coffee drinking. In another study blood pressure increased in caffeine naive subjects, but there were no pressure changes in habitual coffee drinkers.

Recent epidemiology reveals coffee has a negative correlation with blood pressure. For example, the huge Kaiser study of 80,000 persons showed coffee and tea were significantly negatively correlated with blood pressure. A study of 7311 residents in the Minneapolis area produced a negative correlation between coffee and blood pressure. Also a 500 person survey in Italy found a negative correlation. The negative correlation means lower blood pressure is associated with more coffee drinking and higher blood pressure with less coffee consumption. Hence the epidemiology suggests coffee lowers pressure.

An extensive recent review on coffee by Myers concludes with "...caffeine does not cause any persistent increase in blood pressure. Individuals who do not regularly consume caffeine in the diet may experience slight increases in blood pressure when exposed to caffeine, but tolerance rapidly develops, with the blood pressure returning to previous levels."

ALCOHOL

Alcohol has a many faceted effect on cardiovascular disease. One the one hand chronic moderate intake is associated with lower heart disease death rate, but this could well be a spurious relationship (see chapter 10). On the other hand, excessive consumption is associated with increased stroke, congestive heart failure, heart muscle degeneration and hypertension.

The association with hypertension is comparatively new. Before 1977 there was very little data implicating alcohol as a cause of hypertension. Since that time the alcohol-blood pressure link has become unusually strong, having been found in a great many very large epidemiological studies in the U.S and Europe. For example, in the 84,000 person Kaiser Permanente study, alcohol and hypertension were clearly related and this relationship was independent of smoking and obesity. The Intersalt study of 10,000 persons at 52 centers around the world found alcohol intake was significantly and independently related to blood pressure. In the 7300 person Scottish heart health study, alcohol was significantly linked to blood pressure in men but not women. The 9550 person HANES survey found alcohol a significant factor in blood pressure. In the epidemiological surveys, the relationship for alcohol is usually less powerful than for excess body weight, but more powerful than for potassium, calcium and sodium.

Abstinence promptly and consistently lowers blood pressure in chronic and dependent drinkers. In experiments with untreated hypertensives, consumption of 80 grams of alcohol (8 oz of 80 proof alcohol or 28 oz of 12% wine) resulted in gradual increases in both systolic and diastolic pressure. Blood pressure dropped when drinking ceased. In 2 out of 3 studies on normotensives, added alcohol has been shown to have a pressor effect. Many controlled experiments have now demonstrated reduced alcohol results in lower blood pressure.

Animal studies have shown alcohol has complex effects on cell membranes and muscle contraction. Short term acute exposure to alcohol increases cell membrane fluidity, but long term exposure decreases membrane fluidity. Acute short term exposure to alcohol increases cellular sodium, calcium and chloride ion concentrations, whereas potassium, phosphorous and magnesium ion concentrations decrease.

Longer term exposure to alcohol results in greatly increased activity of ATPase, an enzyme responsible for pumping sodium out of cells and potassium into cells. This adaptive response normalizes the sodium and potassium concentrations, but the cellular calcium remains high and the magnesium and phosphorous remains low.

Increased cellular calcium may be a common mechanism for cellular injury by alcohol and other toxic substances. Cell injury by deficiencies or excesses of various substances, including alcohol, invariably results in high concentrations of cellular calcium. A recent study showed high cell calcium concentrations induced protein digesting enzymes to distruct myofibrillar proteins in muscle cells. This could account for the heart muscle degeneration in human and animal alcoholics.

The high cellular calcium concentration in alcoholic rats increases the contractility of smooth muscles and their sensitivity to the following vasopressors: norepinephrine, angiotensin II and vasopressin. This is very likely an important reason why alcohol increases blood pressure.

Altura, in an interesting experiment, discovered alcohol applied to isolated canine cerebral arteries causes spasm of these arteries. The higher the alcohol concentration, the greater the spasm. Altura speculates that the rapid and sometimes sudden behaviour efects of alcohol on humans, such as mental haziness, muscular incoodination, stupor and coma are caused by cerebral artery spasm induced by alcohol.

In summary, the case is very strong implicating alcohol as an important cause of elevated blood pressure. Persons with high blood pressure should eliminate alcohol from their diet. There is much more consistent evidence against alcohol than there is against sodium as a cause of hypertension. Unfortunately the public has not been informed of this effect of alcohol.

SUGAR

The evidence supporting simple sugars as a cause of hypertension is limited. In a controlled experiment, Ahrens reported an average increased blood pressure of 5 mmHg in volunteers given increasing amounts of sucrose (up to 200g per day) for five weeks. Hodges and Rebello compared the short term systolic blood pressure effects of placebo, glucose, fructose, sucrose, galactose or lactose solutions given to normotensive men. An average of 70 grams of sucrose or glucose produced a significant increase in systolic blood pressure two hours later. Diastolic pressure was not influenced. Also, all the sugars, except galactose, significantly decreased short term sodium excretion by varying amounts. Studies on the epidemiology of sugar consumption and hypertension, to my knowledge, have not been done.

The limited animal work supports the human results. Spider monkeys given sodium chloride or sodium chloride plus sucrose had blood pressure increases after eight weeks, but the sodium chloride plus sucrose group had the greatest rise. Rats fed varying amounts of sucrose instead of starch had significantly higher blood pressures. In other work, spontaneously hypertensive and Wistar Kyoto rats had significantly higher blood pressure when fed sucrose and salt. When sucrose was removed from the diet, blood pressure fell but not when only salt was removed. On the other hand Wistar American rats were not sensitive to the salt-sugar regimen.

In summary, the limited animal and human work suggests high sugar consumption may be a factor in hypertension. In terms of risk vs reward it would seem reasonable to recommend lower sugar intake. There are no know risks associated with reduced consumption. The reward may be lower blood pressure, but this is based on limited evidence. Less sugar is consistent with the other recommendations made throughout this book. Less sugar would probably result in some weight loss. The diet would be higher in grains, fruits and vegetables, thereby providing more of the protective potassium, magnesium, fiber and calcium.

REFERENCES

CAFFEINE

Ammon, H. et.al. Adaption of BP to heavy coffee drinking. Br J Clin Pharmacol 15:701-6, 1983

Curatolo, P and Robertson, D. The health consequences of caffeine. Ann Int Med 98:641-653,1983.
Freestone, S. & Ramsay, L. Pressor effect of coffee & cigarettes in hypertensive patients. Clin Sci 63:403s-5s,1982.

Izzo, J. et.al. Age and prior caffeine use alter CV response to coffee. Am J Cardiol 52:769-73, 1983

Myers, M. Effects of Caffeine on Blood Pressure. Arch Intern Med 148:1189-93, 1988.

ALCOHOL

Alderman, E. and Coltart, D. Alcohol and the heart. Brit Med Bull 38:77-80,1982.

Altura, B. et.al. Alcohol induced spasms of cerebral blood vessels. Science 220:331,1983.

Friedman, G. et.al. Alcohol intake and hypertension. Ann Int Med 98:848-849,1983.

Gruchow, H. et.al. Alcohol, nutrient intake and hypertension in US adults. JAMA 253:1567-70, 1985.

Intersalt Cooperative Research Group. Intersalt: an international study. Br Med J 297:319-28, 1988.

Knochel,James, Cardiovascular effects of alcohol. Ann Int Med 98:849-854,1983.

Saunders, J. Alcohol: an important cause of hypertension. Br Med J 294:1045-46, 1987.

Smith, W. et.al. Scottish heart health study. Br Med J 297: 329-30, 1988.

SUGAR

Hodges, R. and Rebello, T., Carbohydrates and blood pressure. Ann Internal Med 98:838-841,1983.

17. SOME FINAL COMMENTS

We have covered a multitude of nutritional factors related to hypertension and cardiovascular disease. They can be classified as either protective or promoting agents. An important strategy to implement for preventing CVD is avoidance of promoters along with increased consumption of protective substances. The promoters to avoid are excessive vitamin D, oxidized cholesterol, saturated fat, total fat, cholesterol, sodium, alcohol, phosphates, sugar, trans fat, animal protein and polished grains. The term "excessive" is important here, since vitamin D, fat, phosphates and sodium are essential for life. This book provides no compeling evidence to eliminate animal protein, but a reasonable case can be made for reducing animal protein to about 6 ounces of meat per day. A much stronger case can be made for using fish as the animal protein, instead of chicken or beef.

In terms of ranking the importance of their promoting properties, I would list vitamin D, oxidized cholesterol, saturated fat, cholesterol, excess weight and total fat first and rank sodium, alcohol, sugar, trans fat, phosphates, polished grains and animal protein further down the list.

Possibly even more important is increased consumption of the protective factors such as potassium, magnesium, fish oils, water soluble fiber, calcium, vitamin B6, vitamin C, vitamin E, copper, zinc, chromium, selenium. Ranking these in terms of protective importance against CVD, I would list fish oils, potassium, magnesium and water soluble fiber first, ranking second would be vitamin B6, calcium, vitamin E, and vitamin C. Further down the list would be chromium, copper, zinc and selenium. The foods providing these nutrients are fish, whole grains, legumes, green leafy vegetables, peppers, cole vegetables, tomatoes, potatoes, tropical fruits, citrus, berries, melons, milk, yogurt, nuts and seeds. I have not listed salad oil or margarine as preferred foods since they are very high in calories with few nutrients and there are no human studies which show they prevent CVD.

Consuming most of your calories from the above foods would make a very remarkable difference in the quantity of protective factors in your diet. Concentrating on protective foods seems to me the most important strategy. Supplements should be considered of secondary importance. If a person is on a nutrient poor diet and does not or will not change, then safe amounts of supplements could be considered.

The average diet in America is 38% fat, 20% polished grain, and 15% sugar, which sums to 73% of our calories. These calories have few nutrients and little fiber. A change to a diet with 20% fat, 5% polished grains and 5% sugar would be much higher in protective nutrients, fiber and much lower in promoters. Certainly the foods to avoid in general are butter, margarine, fats, oils, salad dressing make with fat (almost all of them are), mayonnaise, cookies, cakes, cheeses except for very low fat varieties, cream, fudge, chocolate, fatty meats, ice cream, beer, wine, alcohol, snack foods, pasteries, polished grains, candy and sodas.

Some of you may feel it would be better to be dead than to eliminate all of these foods and deserts. Yes it would be difficult, but I am not talking about complete elimination. I personally feel it can make life unnecessarily difficult and maybe boring. I am taking about significantly reducing the amounts of these foods. The best way to do that for most people is to not buy them at the grocery store routinely, and when you do buy them, buy limited amounts. Also, by purchasing more protective foods you will find your food bill will be reduced.

The above ranking of promoting and protecting factors are my personal evaluations of the scientific evidence. I am sure there are many experts out there who would rank

things differently. My main point in ranking is to emphasize
to the reader that I don't think that every protective factor
or every promoting factor is of equal value. For example, I
happen to think increasing potassium intake is more important
than reducing sodium consumption. But I think doing both is
the most important. Concentrating on having a low sodium
diet is an incomplete strategy. The scientific literature
shows that having high potassium and low sodium is probably
a much better idea. Another example would be fish oil
compared to copper. There is much more powerful and
persuasive evidence on fish oils than there is on copper.
Nevertheless, you can get them both by eating seafoods.

      This, of course is what is so useful about the strategy
of eating more protective foods and avoiding promoting foods.
All of the nutrients and food factors we have covered
will be altered in a very favorable direction by this simple
strategy.

APPENDIX: ATHEROSCLEROSIS and HYPERTENSION

THEORIES OF THE DEVELOPMENT
OF ATHEROSCLEROSIS

Atherosclerosis develops slowly and silently in humans over a long period of time, which makes it impossible to study the natural history of the disease in humans. Animal experiments have never attempted to reproduce the slow, silent development occuring in man. It is assumed the more rapid production of experimental arterial disease in laboratory animals, usually requiring between two months and two years, has many developmental features in common with human atherosclerosis. Since it is not possible to study the natural history in man and the time factor is so different in animals, human atherosclerosis is incompletely understood and will probably remain so for many years.

The first animal experiments which produced atherosclerosis did so by dramatically elevating serum lipid levels in experimental animals. These experiments spawned the infiltration theory of atherosclerosis. The notion was the gruel filled lesions were caused by lipids in the blood filtering through the arteries. It may be true that lipids migrate from the blood through the inner walls of the arteries, but it does not explain many aspects of the disease. This theory predicts a uniform distribution of lesions, but this does not occur. For example, lesions are distributed focally or spot like rather than continuous and they occur much more often in the coronary artery than any other artery. Also, the theory does not account for the complex nature of fibrous plaque with its thickened intima, proliferated smooth muscle cells, connective tissue and cellular debris.

Another early explanation, the incrustation theory, predicted fibrous plaque was caused by clot (thrombus) formation on the arterial wall. Since epithelial and other type cells normally invade thrombi as part of the healing process, it was speculated that this is a natural way to explain fibrous plaque. It is known thrombi often occur in advanced atherosclerosis, but at this time there is no evidence a thrombus exists during the initial stages of lesion development.

A more recent hypothesis is the monoclonal theory of atherosclerosis. It is based on the similarity between a benign muscle tumor and the proliferated smooth muscle in fibrous plaque. There is evidence each lesion is a clone of smooth muscle cells derived from one parent cell, hence the name monoclonal. Indeed fibrous plaque could have some properties in common with a benign tumor, but it does not shed light on other characteristics of atherosclerosis. The distribution of lesions and the accumulation of lipids are not explained by this theory. Also, it doesn't explain most risk factors very well, such as, elevated serum lipids, hypertension, obesity, inactivity and diabetes.

The more recent response to injury hypothesis is widely accepted and explains more experimental findings than the other theories. This concept gained prominence when it was demonstrated mechanical injury to arteries produced the beginning stages of fibrous plaque in animals on normal diets with normal serum lipids. If nothing more is done to the animal, the initial lesions regress, but repeated injury produces irreversible fibrous plaque. Also, initial injury plus elevated serum lipids results in fibrous plaque.

Balloon catheters pulled through monkey, rabbit, dog or rat arteries abrades and denudes the endothelium, exposing the collagen and other connective tissue beneath. The exposed collagen is a powerful inducer of platelet aggregation, therefore shortly after endothelial damage, platelets are found aggregating and adhering to the exposed collagen. Platelet activation and aggregation are critical for lesion development. For example, if the platelets are removed or if platelet stabilizers are given, no fibrous plaque nor the steps leading to it are produced after mechanical injury.

The adhering activated platelets release several important chemicals which are essential for the disease process. One of these is the prostaglandin thromboxane A2 (TXA-2), a powerful promoter of platelet aggregation. The other chemical released is the extraordinarily important platelet derived growth factor (PDGF).

Within three to seven days after the adhered platelets release their chemicals, smooth muscle cells have migrated from the media, through the pores in the internal elastic lamina, into the intima. Under normal circumstances smooth muscle cells are not found in the intima. There is evidence that PDGF causes the smooth muscle cells to migrate from the media to the intima. Tissue culture studies have shown the smooth muscle cells have altered ("modulated") characteristics once they are in the intima for several days. After the smooth muscle cells are "modulated" in the intima, they no longer have the ability to contract, instead they become cells with abilities to divide and make connective tissue. The modulated smooth muscle cells in the intima proliferate and make excessive connective tissue. The proliferation of the smooth muscle cells is stimulated by PDGF. The PDGF, released by the aggregating platelets, plays a decisive role in the development of fibrous plaque by causing smooth muscle proliferation and probably causing their migration from the media to the intima.

It has recently been shown that smooth muscle cells from human fibrous plaque produce large amounts of PDGF, whereas smooth muscle cells from healthy tissue make one fifth as much. This suggests once the disease begins, growth of the lesion becomes self stimulating. Also PDGF down regulates the HDL receptors on fibroblasts. This results in reduced ability for HDL to remove cholesterol from cholesterol laden cells.

If the artery is injured only once and serum lipids are not elevated, then the lesions regress after several months. However, if the artery is subjected to repeated injury, the lesions progress towards full blown fibrous plaque, exhibiting greatly thickened intima, excess connective tissue a lipid deposition under the connective tissue. The fib plaque produced by repeated injury does not regress or

Mechanical devices are not the only means to injure endothelium. In addition, pressure pulse waves going through the arteries, generated by the heart beating 60 to 80 times per minute, cause small amounts of endothelial damage. The fact that pulse waves go through the arteries and not the veins helps to explain why arteries become diseased and veins do not. The locations of the lesions are best explained by the response to injury hypothesis via the pulse trauma. For example, the coronary artery becomes diseased much more often than any other artery and of course it is the first branch off the aorta so it gets the highest pressure pulse waves. Secondly, branching, as found in the coronary artery, causes turbulence in the flow of blood, producing greater impact on the sides of the arteries. This helps to explain why the coronary artery becomes diseased more often than other arteries.

Chemically induced injury produces the same kind of smooth muscle proliferation and fibrous plaque development after repeated exposure. Oxidized cholesterol is an example of a chemical that causes chemical injury of the endothelium. Oxidized cholesterol damages endothelium in tissue and animal studies resulting in atherosclerosis. Chronic exposure to elevated serum cholesterol after mechanical injury also produces non-regressing, lipid infiltrated fibrous plaque. This common finding provides evidence that elevated serum cholesterol causes chronic endothelial damage and/or alteration.

Low density lipoprotein (LDL), the complex of lipid and protein which carries most of the cholesterol in the blood and is positively correlated with increased atherosclerosis in many studies, has been reported to stimulate smooth muscle proliferation and probably the migration of these cells from the media to the intima. In addtion, LDL appears to inhibit the regeneration of healthy endothelium.

There is evidence other circulating chemicals damage the endothelium. Homocystine, a chemical produced when vitamin B6 is in short supply or by persons with a rare inherited disorder called homocystinurea, denudes the endothelium, producing fibrous plaque in laboratory animals and humans with homocystinurea. Viruses or antibody-antigen complexes can also damage endothelium and induce atherosclerosis in laboratory animals.

A number of circulating hormones promote atherosclerosis. Insulin, for instance, is an important risk factor correlated with atherosclerosis and coronary artery disease in many surveys. Whole animal and tissue culture work demonstrates insulin promotes atherosclerosis and stimulates smooth muscle proliferation. Growth hormone is suspected of increasing atherosclerosis and stimulating smooth muscle proliferation. The catacholamines, better known as epinephrine and nor epinephrine, activate platelets and inhibit the growth of endothelium. Possibly this is the link between stress and atherosclerosis, since one of the hormones produced in response to stress is epinephrine.

Important discoveries have been made on the role of macrophages in fibrous plaque development. These scavenger cells of the immune system are present in atherosclerosis at the earliest possible stage, that is, in fatty streak. Lipid filled foam cells, which are universally found in fatty streak, have been shown to be lipid filled macrophages.

The macrophages have unregulated receptors for 'altered' LDL. One way to 'alter' the LDL is to peroxidize the lipids in LDL. Macrophages can ingest 'altered' LDL until they burst. The overingesting, bursting macrophages dump their contents into the 'gruel' of fibrous plaque, very likely forming a major part of the gruel. In addition, macrophages secrete PDGF to stimulate more smooth muscle and fibroblast proliferation. They also secrete fibroblast growth factor and epidermal growth factor.

Macrophages are found in both fatty streak and fibrous plaque. In advanced fibrous plaque they are seen at the leading edge of the necrotic mass of the lesion, where they appear to be dying and dumping their lipid filled contents into the gruel.

HYPERTENSION

Hypertension is closely associated with atherosclerosis, in fact, atherosclerosis is an important factor in hypertension. For example, it has been estimated that a 10% reduction in the diameter of resistance vessels increases peripheral blood flow resistance by 25%. Atherosclerosis is the most important and common cause of blood vessel diameter reduction and increased peripheral resistance is a major factor in hypertension.

Hypertension and atherosclerosis are diseases which feed upon themselves. Not only does atherosclerosis cause hypertension, but hypertension causes atherosclerosis. An important common finding in animals and humans for both diseases is arterial smooth muscle proliferation. Animal hypertension studies have reported smooth muscle proliferation in the arteries is a response to hypertension. Also, greater endothelial denuding and damage occurs in animals with experimental hypertension. With this information, we can add hypertension as another important cause of atherosclerosis made understandable by the response to injury hypothesis.

In its simplest terms, blood pressure is a function of heart output and peripheral resistance of the arteries. When arteries are narrowed due to atherosclerosis or arterial muscle contraction, the resistance to blood flow goes up and so does blood pressure. The increased resistance encourages the heart to increase its output to overcome the resistance, thereby increasing blood pressure further. The increased resistance and output puts a greater strain on the heart which can result in left ventricle enlargement and congestive heart failure.

The autonomic nervous system, endocrine system and kidneys are important regulators of heart output and peripheral resistance. It is beyond the scope of this book to discuss the complex interrelationships of these systems in reglulating blood pressure.

The prevalence of hypertension in the U.S. population depends on the definition of hypertension. If diastolic blood pressure of 90 and above is used as the cut off point, then 25.3% of the population or 56 million people are hypertensive, whereas if 100 and above is used, then the number of people classified as hypertensive drops to 18 million.

Diastolic pressure between 88 and 100 or systolic pressure between 138 and 147 is often labeled borderline or mild hypertension. Some physicians consider these readings to be hypertensive and others do not. In addition to the problem of classifying them, there is also a debate on what to do with these borderline patients. Should they be treated or merely observed? Of course treatment is justified if it can be shown there is good benefit with treatment and little risk.

A 20 year life insurance study of over 4 million persons reported twenty year mortality rates of 20% and 27.2% for normotensives and borderline (88 to 92 mmHg) hypertensives respectively. This is a very moderate but real increase in risk. When the rates are divided by 20, yearly death rates of 1.0% vs 1.36% result, again revealing a very slight increase in death rate.

Within the group of mild hypertensives, there was a wide range of death rates, depending on other risk factors. The Framingham Study has clearly shown a dramatic range of death rates for mild or frank hypertensives, depending on the interaction of other risk factors. For example, a 40 year old man with systolic pressure of 150 and no other major risk factors has a 0.3% chance of dying each year for the succeeding 8 years. A man with the same systolic blood pressure combined with four other risk factors, namely, elevation in serum cholesterol, glucose intolerance, cigarette smoking and electrocardiographically documented left ventricular hypertrophy has a 6.5% chance of dying each year, for a remarkable 2100% increase in risk.

The Framingham data graphically demonstrates hypertension, whether mild or frank, cannot be looked at and evaluated in isolation. A person with mild hypertension and no other risk factors would have a low probability of dying due to his hypertension, hence there would be very little benefit, if any, in treating the mild hypertension with medications. On the other hand, a patient with mild hypertension and one or more of the above risk factors has a significantly higher probability of dying due to his elevated blood pressure, hence there would be better likelihood treatment would be beneficial.

It is difficult to produce unequivocal evidence demonstrating treatment of mild hypertension is beneficial. The U. S. Hypertension, Detection and Followup Program (HDFP) reported a significant decrease in cardiovascular deaths in treated patients with mild hypertension, but a number of experts have pointed out the benefits were more likely due to "more intensive overall medical care" than to the antihypertensive therapy.

The Australian Therapeutic Trial reported a decrease in cardiovascular mortality in treated mild hypertensives, but the decrease was not significant. A curious and potentially disturbing finding in the Australian trial was those persons whose blood pressure dropped below 100 using a placebo had fewer cardiovascular complications than those using drugs to reduce their BP below 100. This illustrates two notions: First, blood pressure often drops spontaneously in the placebo group. In fact, the HDFP trial reported 33% of the patients who were above 95 mm Hg diastolic on the first measurement were below 90 diastolic on their second or succeeding recording. Multiple measurements over a period of time are critical for establishing mild or even frank hypertension.

Second, antihypertensive drug therapy may cause added risks of their own which may not be offset by the benefits of blood pressure reduction. The results of the Multiple Risk Factor Intervention Trial (MRFIT) supports this disturbing possibility. In that study, hypertensives who were aggresively treated with drugs, had a higher death rate than the controls in addition to a pronounced increase in ECG abnormalities.

The above leads directly to the obvious conclusion that hypertensives should first be treated with the lowest risk treatment. The lowest risk treatment is diet and exercise. Weight loss and diets rich in fiber, calcium, magnesium, fish and potassium combined with low fat, low salt and low alcohol should moderate blood pressure in most persons.

REFERENCES

ATHEROSCLEROSIS

Adam, E. et. al. High levels of cytomegalovirus antibody in patients with atherosclerosis. Lancet 2:291-3,1987.

Cathcart, M. et. al. Monocytes and neutrophils oxidize LDL making it cytotoxic. J Leuko Biol 38:341-50,1985.

Hiramatsu, K. et. al. Superoxide initiates oxidation of LDL by human monocytes. Arterio 7:55-60,1987.

Jonasson, L. et. al. Regional accumulations of T cells, macrophages and smooth muscle cells in human atherosclerotic plaque. Arterio 6:131-8,1986.

Kuo, Peter, Lipoproteins, platelets and prostaglandins in atherosclerosis. Am Heart J 102:949-53,1981.

Libby, P. et. al. Production of PDGF-like mitogen by smooth muscle cells. N Engl J Med 318:1493-8,1988.

Mitchinson, M. and Ball, R. Macrophages and atherogenesis. Lancet 2:146-149,1987.

Oppenheimer, M. et. al. Downregulation of HDL receptor by PDGF. Arterio 7:325-32,1987.

Ross, R. Atherosclerosis: A problem of the biology of arterial wall cells and their interactions with blood components. Arterio 1:293-311,1981.

Ross, R. The pathogenesis of atherosclerosis- an update. N Engl J Med 314:488-500,1986.

Ross, R. Platelet-derived growth factor. Ann Rev Med 38: 71-9,1987.

Ruderman, N. and Haudenschild, C. Diabetes as an atherogenic factor. Prog Cardiovas Dis 26:373-409,1984.

Schwartz, S. and Ross, R. Cellular proliferation in atherosclerosis & hypertension. Prog Cardio Dis 26:355-372,1984.

Sims, Frank, A comparison of coronary and internal mammary arteries and implications of the results in the etiology of arteriosclerosis. Am Heart J 105:560-6,1983.

Stout, R. Insulin and atheroma- an update. Lancet 1:1077-79,1987.

Wall, R. and Harker, L., The endothelium and thrombosis. Ann Rev Med 31:361-71,1980.

HYPERTENSION

Kaplan, N., Hypertension: Prevalence, risks and effective therapy. Ann Int Med 98:70s,1983.

ABOUT THE AUTHOR

Ronald S. Smith, B.A. Zoology, University of California, Berkeley, M.S. Chemistry, San Diego State University, Graduate Work in Nutrition, San Jose State University, Graduate Work in Psychology, San Francisco State University, was Professor of Chemistry and Nutrition at Gavilan College for 12 years. Professor Smith was also a Research Chemist at Shell Development's Biological Sciences Research Center. His many publications have appeared in national and international journals. He now devotes full time to research, writing and lecturing nationwide. During the past ten years more than thirty thousand health care professionals have enthusiastically praised his Continuing Education Seminars on nutrition. His various seminars have been on nutrition as it pertains to cardiovascular disease, cancer, brain development and behavior. Since 1974 he has been a student of the scientific literature on nutrition and cardiovascular disease at the Stanford Medical Center and Oregon Health Sciences University. He is a member of the American College of Nutrition, the American Association for the Advancement of Science and the New York Academy of Sciences. He is currently working on two books, one on education and one on nutrition, brain and behavior.